NAPLEX NUGGETS
Your Essential Review of the
Most Highly Testable
Medications from Pharmacy
School

Authored by,
Eric Christianson, Pharm.D., BCPS, BCGP

Copyright and Disclaimer

Cover Illustration and Design Copyright 2017 by: Melissa Christianson

Formatting by: Melissa Christianson

Do you learn best by doing practice questions? Exclusive 35% offer on all NAPLEX practice exams at https://www.meded101.com/naplex/ Use discount code *"**nugget**"* at checkout!

ABOUT THE AUTHOR

Eric Christianson, Pharm.D., BCPS, BCGP is a clinical pharmacist who is passionate about pharmacy education. Eric is the founder of Meded101.com, a website dedicated to providing quality, real world medication education for healthcare professionals. He has been quoted or acknowledged by Pharmacy Times, The Wall Street Journal, American Journal of Nursing, National Association Directors of Nursing, Pharmacy Podcast, and Pharmacy Today.

Please take the time to check out the free resources provided through the website and social media accounts.

Free 6 page PDF at meded101.com - 30 Medication Mistakes

Facebook – https://www.facebook.com/meded101

Twitter - @mededucation101

LinkedIn – Eric Christianson, Pharm.D., BCPS, CGP

INTRODUCTION

I remember what it was like to study for the NAPLEX. Overwhelming doesn't begin to describe the feeling. Where do you start? How do you prioritize and review for this gigantic exam? When I am preparing to take pharmacy exams, I have a very difficult time learning and retaining information from massive review books. I find myself reading for 5-10 minutes and my mind begins to wander, retaining nothing of what I just read. After years of practice and test taking (NAPLEX, BCPS, CGP etc.), I have found that I learn most efficiently by memorizing information in short important bullet points. In this study guide, I have selected the most commonly used medication classes and have provided you with my most highly testable pearls on each class. In this book, I cover over 150 medication classes which includes nearly 400 medications! I have created bullet points which will help you review more efficiently and not waste your limited study time. This resource is not intended to be a package insert for every medication, but rather a way to try to prioritize your study process and understand the major "nuggets" of information that you must know to help you pass the NAPLEX. The intent is to give you a brief, incredibly helpful review of the most important medications you will likely be tested on the NAPLEX exam. I truly hope this book helps you pass the NAPLEX the first time!

Table of Contents

1ST Generation Antipsychotics (Typicals)

Example: Haloperidol (Haldol), Perphenazine, Chlorpromazine, Fluphenazine, Prochlorperazine (Compazine), Thioridazine

Mechanism of Action: Blocks dopamine receptors

NAPLEX Nuggets:
- Common Uses: Schizophrenia, Bipolar disorder, (off label - dementia related behaviors like aggression, hallucinations or delusions)
- Memorable Side Effects: Sedation, fall risk, orthostatic BP changes, EPS, metabolic syndrome
- Haloperidol is the classic first generation antipsychotic and has a very high rate of EPS (movement disorder side effects) which is a major reason why atypicals (2nd generation) are generally preferred
- Usually higher doses are required for younger patients with schizophrenia and/or bipolar disorder while lower doses can and should be used in the elderly
- Remember with antipsychotic medications that they block dopamine and can exacerbate conditions where there is a shortage of dopamine like Parkinson's disorder (remember that we use dopamine to treat Parkinson's – i.e. carbidopa/levodopa)
- Sedation, orthostatic hypotension, movement disorder side effects can all increase the risk of falls especially in our elderly patients
- NMS (neuroleptic malignant syndrome) is a very rare but very serious complication with antipsychotic medications; a few symptoms of NMS include: fever, hyperreflexia, confusion, delirium, tremor
- Antipsychotics increase risk of metabolic syndrome (diabetes, elevated lipids, weight gain, etc.) – it is important to periodically monitor for this, especially in younger patients with schizophrenia and/or bipolar who may be likely to require long term use of higher doses

- Anticholinergic effects are possible as well with antipsychotics, dry eyes, dry mouth, exacerbation of urinary retention (i.e. BPH), constipation (SLUD – can't salivate, lacrimate, urinate or defecate)
- Antipsychotics can contribute to QTc prolongation, which can be especially problematic in patients who are already at risk (i.e. on antiarrhythmic medications)
- Chlorpromazine sometimes used for N/V or intractable hiccups
- Compazine commonly used as antiemetic

2-Azetidinone – Lipid Reducer

Example: Ezetimibe (Zetia)

Mechanism of Action: Inhibits intestinal absorption of cholesterol

NAPLEX Nuggets:
- Common Uses: Elevated cholesterol, particularly LDL
- Memorable Side Effects: Overall usually well tolerated, low risk of diarrhea, myopathy (especially when used in combo with statins)
- May be used in combination with a statin
- Pretty well tolerated when used alone, but not nearly as potent at reducing LDL as statins
- Still fairly expensive at this time (and don't get that great of LDL reduction)
- Can possibly increase risk of rhabdomyolysis when added to statin therapy, so need to watch out for muscle pain/soreness etc.
- Once daily dosing is nice

2ND Generation Antipsychotics (Atypicals)

Example: Aripiprazole (Abilify), Quetiapine (Seroquel), Risperidone (Risperdal), Clozapine (Clozaril), Ziprasidone (Geodon), Olanzapine (Zyprexa)

Mechanism of Action: Blocks dopamine receptors

NAPLEX Nuggets:

- Common Uses: Schizophrenia, bipolar disorder, depression, dementia related behaviors like aggression, hallucinations, delusions (off-label)
- Aripiprazole can be used in patients who have failed traditional monotherapy like SSRI's for depression (usually this is at low doses)
- Usually higher doses are required for younger patients with schizophrenia and/or bipolar disorder while lower doses can and should be used in the elderly
- Remember with antipsychotic medications that they block dopamine and can exacerbate conditions where there is a shortage of dopamine like Parkinson's disorder (remember that we use dopamine to treat Parkinson's – i.e. carbidopa/levodopa); quetiapine may have least risk of exacerbating Parkinson's
- Long term use of dopamine blockers can cause the development of tardive dyskinesia (often referred to as TD)
- Sedation, orthostatic hypotension, movement disorder side effects can all increase the risk of falls especially in our elderly patients
- EPS (movement side effects) generally more common with the 1st generation antipsychotics
- NMS (neuroleptic malignant syndrome) is a very rare but very serious complication with antipsychotic medications; a few symptoms of NMS include: fever, hyperreflexia, confusion, delirium, tremor

- Antipsychotics increase risk of metabolic syndrome (diabetes, elevated lipids, weight gain etc.) – it is important to periodically monitor for this, especially in younger patients with schizophrenia and/or bipolar who may be likely to require long term use of higher doses (olanzapine and clozapine considered worse for this adverse effect)
- Can potentially cause hyperprolactinemia (prolactin stimulates the production of breast milk)
- Anticholinergic effects are possible as well with antipsychotics, dry eyes, dry mouth, exacerbation of urinary retention (i.e. BPH), constipation (SLUD – can't salivate, lacrimate, urinate or defecate)
- Antipsychotics can contribute to QTc prolongation, which can be especially problematic in patients who are already at risk (i.e. on antiarrhythmic medications)
- Clozapine can cause life threatening agranulocytosis (drop in white blood cell count/neutrophils)

5-Alpha Reductase Inhibitors

Example: Dutasteride (Avodart), Finasteride (Proscar, Propecia)

Mechanism of Action: Inhibits 5-alpha reductase which results in less dihydrotestosterone

NAPLEX Nuggets:
- Common Uses: BPH, baldness (finasteride)
- Memorable Side Effects: Impotence, weakness
- Not for immediate relief of acute urinary retention due to BPH!
- Takes weeks to months for clinical benefit
- Pretty well tolerated usually with impotence being most common
- Keep an eye out for drugs that exacerbate BPH (anticholinergics)

ACE Inhibitors

Example: Benazepril (Lotensin), Lisinopril (Zestril), Ramipril (Altace), Enalapril/Enalaprilat - injectable (Vasotec), Captopril (Capoten), Fosinopril (Monopril), Quinapril (Accupril), Moexipril (Univasc)

Mechanism of Action: Inhibits the angiotensin converting enzyme. This prevents the production of angiotensin 2; less angiotensin 2 equates to less vasoconstriction, and lower blood pressure

NAPLEX Nuggets:
- Common Uses: Hypertension
- Common Side Effects: Cough, kidney impairment, low blood pressure, and hyperkalemia
- ACE Inhibitors are notoriously known for causing a dry chronic cough
- Angiotensin Receptor Blockers (ARBs) are the cousins to the ACE Inhibitors, and are the first line substitute to a patient who has had a cough with an ACE Inhibitor
- ACE inhibitors can exacerbate (but also can be kidney protective!) kidney impairment as well as contribute to acute renal failure especially in patients who are already on other potential renal toxic medications (i.e. diuretics, NSAIDs etc.) even though in conditions like heart failure, diuretics and ACE Inhibitors are often used together – monitor for a rising creatinine, falling GFR
- Captopril rarely used as it requires frequent dosing
- ACE Inhibitors are a classic cause of elevated potassium levels; if your patient has hyperkalemia, you must make sure the ACE Inhibitor has been addressed
- In some cases, African Americans may not respond to ACE Inhibitors as well as other ethnicities
- A common mistake I've seen clinicians make is using an ACE Inhibitor with an ARB; this is generally not recommended

- Compelling Indications: ACE Inhibitors are frequently used in patients with hypertension and a history of diabetes, stroke, CAD, CKD, and CHF

Acetylcholinesterase inhibitors

Example: Donepezil (Aricept), Galantamine (Razadyne), Rivastigmine (Exelon)

Mechanism of Action: Inhibits acetylcholinesterase which increases acetylcholine in the CNS

NAPLEX Nuggets:

- Common Uses: Alzheimer's dementia
- Memorable Side Effects: GI (N/V/D), weight loss, insomnia
- Remember opposite effects of anticholinergics
- One of the common drug causes of weight loss in the elderly
- Donepezil usually dosed at night (to minimize GI risk, but rarely can cause insomnia)
- Likely will NOT reverse dementia symptoms, but used to delay progression (slow down patients from getting worse)
- Dementia medications in general can contribute to behavioral changes (good or bad)
- Rivastigmine has a patch formulation (expensive however)

Adrenergic Agonist - Systemic

Example: Dopamine, Dobutamine

Mechanism of Action: Stimulates adrenergic and dopamine receptors

NAPLEX Nuggets:
- Common Uses: shock, heart failure
- Memorable Side Effects: BP, Pulse changes, N/V, arrhythmia
- At low doses may actually cause renal vasodilation
- At higher doses more likely to act like epinephrine (stimulates heart and vasoconstriction – increase pulse/BP)
- Usually volume replacement is first in kidney failure, but this may be used adjunct in certain situations for shock

Alpha and Beta agonist (Intravenous)

Example: Norepinephrine (Levophed)

Mechanism of Action: Stimulates alpha and beta receptors leading to increased BP, pulse

NAPLEX Nuggets:
- Common Uses: Treatment of shock (severe hypotension)
- Memorable Side Effects: hypertension, arrhythmias, anxiety
- Clamps down on vessels causing an increase in BP
- Chest pain possible due to reduced blood flow through the heart
- Boxed warning for extravasation

Alpha-Blockers

Example: Doxazosin (Cardura), Terazosin (Hytrin), Tamsulosin (Flomax), Prazosin (Minipress)

Mechanism of Action: Blocks alpha receptors causing smooth muscle relaxation, vasodilation and opening of the ureter

NAPLEX Nuggets:

- Common Uses: BPH, urinary obstruction, hypertension
- Memorable Side Effects: Low BP, dizziness
- Non-selective alpha blocker can be used for both hypertension and BPH
- Risk of orthostasis higher with a non-selective alpha blockers
- In the case of worsening urinary retention due to BPH and initiation of these agents, be sure to assess if your patient is on anticholinergic medications (diphenhydramine, TCA's etc.)
- Usually dosed at night to minimize the risk of orthostasis
- Tamsulosin is more selective for bladder (generally not used for hypertension)
- Prazosin used off label for nightmares

Alpha-Glucosidase Inhibitors
Example: Acarbose (Precose), Meglitol (Glyset)

Mechanism of Action: Blocks breakdown of complex carbohydrates in the GI tract and prevents absorption thus reducing blood sugar

NAPLEX Nuggets:
- Dosed three times per day which limits its use
- High incidence of GI adverse effects which patients don't like (also limits their use)
- Need to be taken with meals
- Target is post prandial glucose levels
- Very important to educate patients that oral glucose needs to be used in the event of hypoglycemic episode – the drug blocks the breakdown of sucrose, so the hypoglycemia may not improve

Aminoglycoside, Antibiotic

Example: Gentamicin, Tobramycin

Mechanism of Action: Blocks bacterial protein synthesis, binds to 30S and 50S subunits

NAPLEX Nuggets:

- Common Uses: Gram negative bacteria; UTI's, sepsis, skin infections
- Memorable Side Effects: CNS changes, diarrhea, kidney impairment, changes in hearing
- Kidney function monitoring is critical – classic nephrotoxic drug
- Monitoring of drug levels important
- Usual trough target is less than 2mcg/mL
- Ototoxicity (ear) is more likely with prolonged use
- Peak sample usually drawn 30 minutes after infusion complete and trough right before next dose
- Ophthalmic dosage forms available for bacterial pink eye

Analgesic/Antipyretic (non-NSAID)

Example: Acetaminophen (Tylenol)

Mechanism of Action: Inhibits prostaglandins in the CNS and may also block pain impulses

NAPLEX Nuggets:

- One of the safest oral medications in the elderly for pain
- First line for osteoarthritis
- Dosing of 10-15 mg/kg/dose in pediatrics
- Typically used in pregnancy first line for pain/headaches, etc. if a medication is necessary
- 4 gram max (possibly 3 gram in elderly/over the counter use)
- Often found in combo with over the counter and prescription medications; cough and cold products, Vicodin, Percocet etc. (be sure patients are well educated on this to avoid accidental overdose)
- Liver toxicity extremely rare at recommended doses, usually problem occurs when accidental or intentional overdose happens

- Acetylcysteine is antidote for acetaminophen overdose
- Usually well tolerated with few drug interactions

Androgen

Example: Testosterone (Androgel, Androderm)

Mechanism of Action: Testosterone hormone -responsible for development of male sex organs, and causes muscle growth

NAPLEX Nuggets:

- Common Uses: Testosterone deficiency, metastatic breast cancer
- Memorable Side Effects: Gynecomastia, hypertension, acne, mood changes
- Drug of abuse in sports (increases muscle mass, etc.)
- Controlled substance – schedule 3 for above reason
- Testosterone can "amp" you up…think of "Roid Rage" – increased BP, irritability, mood swings, anger, etc.
- Risk of DVT a possibility (rare)
- Increase in PSA and possible impotence especially with prolonged use

Anesthetic, Sedative (Miscellaneous)

Example: Propofol (Diprivan)

Mechanism of Action: Possible agonist activity on GABA and blockade of NMDA

NAPLEX Nuggets:
- Common Uses: Anesthesia (intubated/ICU type patients)
- Memorable Side Effects: Hypotension, respiratory apnea, elevated triglycerides, respiratory acidosis
- Infusion contains lipids (explains the possibility for elevated triglycerides)
- Rare risk for anaphylaxis
- Can be riskier in patients who already have lower blood pressure
- Very fast onset (less than 1 minute)

Antiarrhythmic – Class 3

Example: Amiodarone (Cardarone)

Mechanism of Action: Multiple mechanisms including affecting sodium/potassium and calcium channels, as well as potentially having beta and alpha blocking activity

NAPLEX Nuggets:

- The usual goal in atrial fibrillation is to control the rate of the heart with beta-blockers or calcium channel blockers (remember only the calcium channel blockers that act on the heart and need to be monitored for pulse – diltiazem and verapamil); Amiodarone is used to control the heart rhythm, not rate, and is usually used second
- Unique in that it has a very long half-life – it takes about 40-55 days for half of the drug to be eliminated
- Thyroid function needs to be monitored
- Respiratory function should be monitored as amiodarone can cause pulmonary fibrosis (it has a black box warning)
- Liver function needs to be monitored as it has a boxed warning for liver toxicity as well
- Classic drug interaction with digoxin – end result is that digoxin concentrations can be significantly elevated when amiodarone is started or increased

Antiarrhythmic, Cardiac Glycoside

Example: Digoxin (Digitek, Lanoxin)

Mechanism of Action: Inhibition of sodium/potassium ATPase, increased contractility, suppression of the AV node

NAPLEX Nuggets:
- Common Uses: Atrial fibrillation, heart failure
- Memorable Side Effects: nausea, vomiting, bradycardia, cognitive changes, weight loss, visual changes (usually at very high levels)
- Classic symptoms of digoxin toxicity involve GI side effects, bradycardia, cognitive changes and weight loss
- Often providers will use hold parameters in healthcare settings to prevent pulse from going to low (i.e. hold digoxin if pulse is less than 60)
- Used for rate control in AFib (may be used instead of beta-blocker or CCB if patient has low blood pressure)
- Digoxin is cleared by the kidney; it can accumulate and be much more likely to cause toxicity in the elderly as patients tend to have worse kidney function as they age
- Higher doses are usually used in atrial fibrillation as compared to heart failure (higher target concentration)
- Upper limit of normal for a digoxin level is usually considered 2 ng/mL
- Patients with low levels of potassium are at greater risk of toxicity, it is really important to assess potassium as many patients on digoxin may also be on diuretics (usually for heart failure) that can deplete potassium
- Benefit for morbidity only in CHF
- Antidote: Digoxin Immune Fab (Digibind or DigiFab)

Antibiotic, Antimycobacterials

Example: Rifampin (Rifadin)

Mechanism of Action: Inhibits bacterial RNA synthesis

NAPLEX Nuggets:
- Common Uses: TB, augmentation in MRSA/osteomyelitis
- Memorable Side Effects: LFT's increased, GI, rash
- CYP enzyme inducer – notorious for drug interactions like warfarin (causes lower INR when initiated)
- MRSA activity

Antibiotic, Glycopeptide

Example: Vancomycin (Vancocin)

Mechanism of Action: Inhibits bacterial cell wall synthesis

NAPLEX Nuggets:
- Common Uses: MRSA (methicillin resistant Staph. aureus), orally can be used to treat C. diff
- Memorable Side Effects: hypotension, flushing, red man syndrome (pretty rare now), given orally – GI adverse effects
- Red man syndrome possible if infused too quickly
- If red man syndrome happens, should be able to slow infusion rate to help treat
- Trough concentration and kidney function may be important to help guide dosing
- Drug of choice for methicillin resistant Staph. aureus (MRSA)
- You should never see this medication taken orally (one exception is a GI infection like C. Diff) – it has poor oral absorption into the blood circulation through the GI tract'
- 10-20 is target trough level – higher end for more serious/life threatening infections

Antibiotic, Lincosamide

Example: Clindamycin (Cleocin)

Mechanism of Action: Inhibits bacterial protein synthesis

NAPLEX Nuggets:

- Common Uses: Skin, bone, joint infections
- Memorable Side Effects: GI side effects, colitis (C. diff risk), metallic taste
- Possible alternative for patients who need antibiotic prophylaxis undergoing dental procedures who can't tolerate or have an allergy to penicillin antibiotics
- One of the common antibiotics that may contribute to C. diff development (quinolones, broader spectrum cephalosporin's, and penicillin's may contribute as well)
- Has some activity again MRSA (methicillin resistant Staph. aureus) where penicillin antibiotics would not be effective
- Frequent administration is kind of a nuisance – usually 3-4 times per day
- Recommended to give with a full glass of water to minimize esophageal ulceration risk
- Topical formulation also available (acne or bacterial vaginosis)

Antibiotic, Miscellaneous

Example: Metronidazole (Flagyl)

Mechanism of Action: Interferes with bacterial DNA and can inhibit protein synthesis

NAPLEX Nuggets
- Common Uses: C. diff, H. pylori, anaerobic infections (gut infections), bacterial vaginosis, Trichomoniasis, Antiprotozoal, Amoebas
- Memorable Side Effects: GI side effects, metallic taste
- Usual first line treatment for C. diff (oral vancomycin is another common option)
- Can be utilized for anaerobic bacteria (Gut infections like diverticulitis, peritonitis)
- Commonly used in combo in treatment of Helicobacter pylori (H. pylori is a common cause of GI ulcers)
- NO ALCOHOL with this medication – causes disulfiram reaction
- Notorious interaction with warfarin via CYP2C9 – increases INR
- IV and PO available

Antibiotic, Miscellaneous

Example: Nitrofurantoin (Macrobid)

Mechanism of Action: Inhibits bacterial protein synthesis, metabolism, DNA, RNA, and cell wall synthesis

NAPLEX Nuggets:
- Common Uses: Urinary tract infection
- Memorable Side Effects: GI, CNS (more likely in elderly), neuropathy(rare), pulmonary distress (rare)
- Have use reassessed if patient has kidney disease at what CrCl is a little controversial (contraindicated for sure <30)
- May discolor urine – be sure to educate patients on this (brown/orange color)
- Rare adverse effect of respiratory issues
- Generally not first line in the elderly for UTI's
- Category B (so potential option in pregnancy)

Antibiotic, Miscellaneous

Example: Trimethoprim/sulfamethoxazole (Bactrim)

Mechanism of Action: Sulfamethoxazole inhibits bacterial folic acid production which trimethoprim essentially does the same via a different mechanism

NAPLEX Nuggets:
- Common Uses: UTI, URI's, PCP (common in HIV patients)
- Memorable Side Effects: GI, rash, CNS changes
- Very common treatment for UTI
- Sulfa allergy is common in many patients! Look out!
- Major drug interaction with warfarin (increases INR)
- Has some activity against MRSA
- Trimethoprim can increase risk for hyperkalemia in patients on ACEI's, ARB's, Potassium supplements, and Potassium Sparing Diuretics

Anticholinergic, Urinary

Example: Oxybutynin (Ditropan), Tolterodine (Detrol), Darifenacin (Enablex), Solifenacin (Vesicare)

Mechanism of Action: Blocks muscarinic receptors (anticholinergic) in the bladder which increases urine volume in the bladder and potentially decreases frequency/urge

NAPLEX Nuggets:
- Common Uses: Overactive bladder, bladder spasms
- Memorable Side Effects: Anticholinergic effects possible (i.e. can't spit, see, pee or poop - dry mouth, dry eyes, urinary retention, constipation)
- Anticholinergic effects (oxybutynin is highly anticholinergic and less selective for the bladder so risk of CNS effects may be increased as well)
- Be sure to assess if the medication is working for incontinence/frequency – many patients don't benefit
- Keep an eye out for patients on diuretics and if urinary frequency is the major issue, make sure that they are minimized if possible (not always possible to reduce diuretics with CHF history, etc.)
- Frequency can be especially problematic in patients who have an active social life as well as night when trying to sleep
- Oxybutynin has a patch formulation available (usually dosed twice weekly)

Anticholinergics (Systemic)

Example: Atropine, Diphenhydramine (Benadryl), Hydroxyzine (Atarax, Vistaril), Benztropine (Cogentin), Dicyclomine (Bentyl), Hyoscyamine (Levsin), Scopolamine (Transderm-Scop), Trihexyphenidyl (Artane), Doxylamine

Mechanism of Action: Blocks acetylcholine in the parasympathetic system which decreases secretions and increases cardiac output

NAPLEX Nuggets:
- Common Uses: sleep, allergies, motion sickness, itching, reduce salivary secretions (atropine drops); pre-op as well as end of life, bradycardia (atropine), treatment of GI spasms (Dicyclomine), Parkinson's, treatment of EPS (from antipsychotics)
- Memorable Side Effects: Highly anticholinergic (can't spit, see, pee, poop)
- Newer antihistamines preferred for allergies (loratadine, cetirizine etc.)
- Oral drops (atropine) used frequently in hospice to decrease excessive salivation
- Can cause significant urinary retention (watch out in BPH)
- Psychotic type symptoms are possible with high enough doses ("mad as a hatter")
- EKG monitoring critical if using for bradycardia – atropine
- Benztropine and trihexyphenidyl used for EPS/Parkinson's versus other anticholinergics (sometimes Benadryl)
- Diphenhydramine/doxylamine commonly found in many OTC sleep aids, cough and cold medicines etc.
- If diarrhea is an issue associated with a patient's IBS, the anticholinergic effect (dicyclomine also can help with

spasms) of constipation can certainly contribute to the patient's benefit

- Classic Prescribing Cascade examples:
    - Anticholinergic then BPH meds added – (i.e. tamsulosin, finasteride)
    - Anticholinergic then artificial tears or artificial saliva
    - Anticholinergic then constipation medications

Anticoagulant, Factor 10A Inhibitor

Example: Rivaroxaban (Xarelto), Apixaban (Eliquis), Edoxaban (Savaysa)

Mechanism of Action: Inhibits clotting factor 10A

NAPLEX Nuggets:
- Common Uses: Prevention of stroke in patients with Atrial Fibrillation, DVT/PE prophylaxis or treatment
- Memorable Side Effects: Bleeding
- Gaining popularity against warfarin
- Less risk of drug interaction as well as patients do NOT need to do routine INR's
- With bleed risk being the major side effect, hemoglobin (CBC) is important to monitor
- Major use of this medication is to prevent or treat blood clots (DVT, PE, Stroke)
- Expensive $$ is the major downside versus warfarin

Anticoagulant, Low Molecular Weight Heparin

Example: Enoxaparin (Lovenox)

Mechanism of Action: Primarily inhibits factor 10A clotting factor (anticoagulant)

NAPLEX Nuggets:
- Common Uses: Used in MI, DVT prophylaxis, DVT treatment
- Memorable Side Effects: Bleed risk, thrombocytopenia (rare)
- Bleeding risk is the major adverse effect that needs to be monitored with any medication that inhibits clotting factors
- It is a heparin based product (low molecular weight heparin) so risk of heparin induced thrombocytopenia is there, but much lower than heparin
- Checking INR's with Enoxaparin is not necessary; weight based dosing
- Platelets and Hemoglobin are two important monitoring parameters (part of a CBC)
- Often patients are bridged to warfarin with orders to start warfarin, and follow INR and when INR is 2 or greater, then discontinue enoxaparin
- Dose adjustments for CrCl less than 30
- Significantly higher dose of enoxaparin recommended for treatment of blood clot (DVT) versus prevention
- Injection only is a downside and why patients are often transitioned to an oral anticoagulant

Anticoagulant, Thrombin inhibitor

Example: Dabigatran (Pradaxa)

Mechanism of Action: Direct thrombin inhibitor which leads to prevention of blood clots

NAPLEX Nuggets:
- Common Uses: Atrial fibrillation, DVT
- Memorable Side Effects: Bleeding
- Bleed risk! Monitor for bruising, low hemoglobin, blood in stools, nose bleeds etc.
- There is a reversal agent available! (expensive)
- Twice daily dosing makes it a little inconvenient
- Be aware to have provider assess for dose adjustment in patients with CKD
- Alternative to warfarin and routine INR is not necessary
- GI bleed risk high in patients >75 y/o
- Avoid/minimize use of medications that can increase bleed risk (NSAIDs are classic example)

Anticoagulants - Heparin

Example: Heparin

Mechanism of Action: Primarily inactivates thrombin, also may have effects on other clotting factors

NAPLEX Nuggets:
- Common Uses: Treatment and prevention of clots, also used in PCI, and to prevent clotting/flush IV lines
- Memorable Side Effects: Bleeding, thrombocytopenia, HIT (rare)
- Bleed risk is top monitoring parameter
- Risk of thrombocytopenia (heparin induced thrombocytopenia – "HIT") – platelets are very important to monitor
- Used to flush IV lines (prevent clotting)
- Many concentrations available (scary for medication error risk)
- Protamine is antidote

Anti-dementia, NMDA Antagonist

Example: Memantine (Namenda)

Mechanism of Action: Blocks NMDA receptors which reduces the activity of glutamate (an excitatory amino acid that has activity in the CNS and potentially contributes to Alzheimer's)

NAPLEX Nuggets:

- Common Uses: Alzheimer's dementia (moderate to severe)
- Memorable Side Effects: Changes in behavior, worsening confusion, dizziness
- Remember that medications used for dementia only delay the progression; i.e. they do NOT reverse dementia and at best help slow the process of getting worse
- Memantine has dose adjustments in kidney disease, so keep an eye out for our patients who may have worsening kidney function (rising creatinine) as the drug may begin to accumulate
- There is both an extended release and immediate release product available now
- Memantine has a different mechanism of action from other dementia medications (i.e. donepezil etc.) so it can be used in combination

Antidepressant - Miscellaneous

Example: Bupropion (Wellbutrin, Zyban)

Mechanism of Action: Not well understood, thought to increase dopamine/norepinephrine (NOT serotonin)

NAPLEX Nuggets:
- Common Uses: Depression, smoking cessation
- Memorable Side Effects: Insomnia/activating, increases seizure risk, GI side effects
- Generally not used first line for depression unless a patient is also looking to stop smoking
- Tends to be more activating (insomnia adverse effect)
- Less risk of reduced libido compared to SSRI's
- Avoid if possible in a patient with a seizure history

Antidepressant, Alpha-2 Antagonist

Example: Mirtazapine (Remeron)

Mechanism of Action: Blocks alpha 2 which increases norepinephrine and serotonin; also antagonist at certain serotonin receptors and H1 receptors

NAPLEX Nuggets:
- Common Uses: Depression, insomnia, anorexia
- Memorable Side Effects: sedation, weight gain (can be good or bad), CNS effects
- Can be used to help with sleep (tends to be more sedating at lower doses) – H1 blocking effects
- Weight gain can be a problem in younger patients, but can be a positive in frail elderly
- Not likely to be beneficial as needed except possibly for insomnia (takes weeks to work for depression or anxiety)

Antidepressant, Serotonin Modulator, Miscellaneous

Example: Trazodone (Desyrel), Nefazodone (Serzone)

Mechanism of Action: Inhibits reuptake of serotonin, but differs from SSRI's in that it has blocking activity on H1 and alpha 1 receptors (H1 blocking activity gives this medication its sedative properties)

NAPLEX Nuggets:
- Common Uses: Sleep, depression
- Memorable Side Effects: Sedation, dizziness, orthostasis
- While it is usually classified as an antidepressant, trazodone at lower doses is most frequently used for insomnia
- Usually the antidepressant benefits of trazodone are seen at higher doses
- Must educate patients on its sedative properties and risk of driving, etc.
- Trazodone can be used "prn" or as needed for sleep, but you should never see it used as needed for depression as it usually takes significant time (like SSRI's) for the antidepressant effect to begin
- Keep an eye out for postural hypotension (dizziness upon rising) especially in our elderly patients and those already on blood pressure lowering medications – if you remember from the mechanism of action above, it does have alpha blocking activity
- Can contribute to dry mouth, be on the lookout for patients who complain about this or are using saliva substitute medications (example: Biotene)
- Nefazodone rarely used due to liver toxicity issues

Anti-diabetic agent, Sulfonylurea

Example: Glipizide (Glucotrol), Glyburide (Diabeta), Glimepiride (Amaryl), Chlorpropamide

Mechanism of Action: Stimulates pancreatic cells to produce/release insulin

NAPLEX Nuggets:
- Memorable Side Effects: Hypoglycemia, weight gain
- Via its mechanism of action, whenever you increase insulin, hypoglycemia is of highest concern
- Be attentive to appetite changes or new diabetes medications and monitor for hypoglycemia
- Often you will see blood sugars bottom out in the early morning when awakening (sleeping is generally the longest period of time when you don't eat)
- Elderly can be especially at risk for hypoglycemia (chlorpropamide on Beer's list)
- Weight gain can be problematic in type 2 patients as many likely struggle with metabolic syndrome/weight control already
- Chlorpropamide can cause SIADH (rarely used due to this and Beer's list designation)
- Glipizide generally preferred in elderly

Antidiabetic, Biguanide

Example: Metformin (Glucophage)

Mechanism of Action: Decreases hepatic glucose production

NAPLEX Nuggets:
- Common Uses: Diabetes
- Memorable Side Effects: N/V/D most common, B12 deficiency possible, lactic acidosis (very rare, more common in patients with poor kidney function)
- Doesn't stimulate production of insulin which is why it is not likely to cause hypoglycemia when used alone
- Metformin is the first line medication for type 2 diabetes
- Metformin is contraindicated in patients with poor kidney function (serum creatinine >1.4 in females and >1.5 in males); if you know a patient has a history of chronic kidney disease (CKD) make sure use of this medication is reassessed – ***labeling becoming less restrictive possibly use down to 30 mls/min
- The risk of lactic acidosis increases as this medication is used in the elderly and those with poor kidney function
- The most common side effect of metformin is GI upset – be on the lookout for patient complaints of this adverse effect and new medication use like PPI's (omeprazole etc.) or other medications that are used to relieve stomach symptoms
- Administration with a meal is recommended and can really help minimize GI upset
- Metformin tends to not cause weight gain compared to other diabetes medications which is nice considering that many of our type 2 diabetes patients are overweight

Antidiabetic, DDP-4 inhibitor

Example: Sitagliptin (Januvia), Linagliptan (Tradjenta), Saxagliptan (Onglyza)

Mechanism of Action: Inhibits DPP-4 which increases incretin levels (incretin increases insulin and decreases glucagon in the body and also might help patients' stomachs "feel full")

NAPLEX Nuggets:
- Common Uses: Diabetes (type 2)
- Memorable Side Effects: GI (usually pretty well tolerated); pancreatitis and cardiovascular concerns exist, but are rare
- Usually fairly well tolerated, once daily dosing is nice for a diabetes medication
- Watch out for dose adjustment and accumulation in CKD
- Usually second or third choice following metformin and/or sulfonylurea in the management of type 2 diabetes (dependent upon how much A1C lowering is necessary)
- Can be found in combination pill with metformin

Antidiabetic, Thiazolidinedione (TZD)

Example: Pioglitazone (Actos), Rosiglitazone (Avandia)

Mechanism of Action: Improves tissue sensitivity to insulin leading to a reduction in blood glucose

NAPLEX Nuggets:

- Common Uses: Diabetes (type 2)
- Memorable Side Effects: Edema, CHF exacerbation, possible elevations in LFT's (rare)
- Usually dosed once daily which is nice (Actos)
- If you see a patient on furosemide or other medications that might indicate CHF, a TZD is not a good choice as it can worsen edema and exacerbate CHF
- Monitor for low blood sugar risk, especially in patients on sulfonylureas (i.e. glipizide) or insulins
- A1C will be important to monitor in any patient on diabetes medications
- Goal is to keep A1C low and minimize risk of hypoglycemia (this will help decrease risk of diabetes complications like neuropathy, retinopathy, worsening kidney function etc.)

Antidiarrheal

Example: Loperamide (Imodium)

Mechanism of Action: Acts on opioid receptors on intestines and slows peristalsis (GI movement)

NAPLEX Nuggets:
- Common Uses: Diarrhea
- Memorable Side Effects: Constipation, abdominal pain
- Over-the-counter availability
- Make sure to have patients who use this chronically on their own assessed for other problems (IBS, infection, adverse effects of other medications etc.)
- Can be used as needed
- Not a controlled substance because it only works on opioid receptors in the gut

Antidiarrheal - Miscellaneous

Example: Diphenoxylate/atropine (Lomotil)

Mechanism of Action: Diphenoxylate inhibits GI motility (atropine is highly anticholinergic and really intended to minimize risk of drug abuse)

NAPLEX Nuggets:
- Common Uses: Diarrhea
- Memorable Side Effects: Pretty well tolerated - Abdominal distress, possibility of anticholinergic effects, but not very likely as atropine dose is very low
- Controlled substance
- Can be used as needed
- Be sure patients who are on this chronically have been assessed for medical and possible medication causes of chronic diarrhea

Antiemetic, GI Prokinetic

Example: Metoclopramide (Reglan)

Mechanism of Action: Blocks dopamine and serotonin receptors (in CRZ – chemoreceptor zone, lends to relief of nausea/vomiting)

NAPLEX Nuggets:
- Common Uses: Gastroparesis (often caused by diabetes), nausea/vomiting
- Memorable Side Effects: Extrapyramidal symptoms, sedation, gynecomastia, hyperprolactinemia
- Has dopamine blocking activity like antipsychotics, so can cause movement disorders like EPS and tardive dyskinesia
- As above with dopamine blocking activity, not a great choice in a patient with a preexisting movement disorder (i.e. Parkinson's)
- Most commonly used for gastroparesis (slow moving GI tract) – be on the lookout for anticholinergic medications which can worsen gastroparesis
- Usually dosed multiple times per day (3-4)

Antiemetic, Miscellaneous

Example: Meclizine (Antivert)

Mechanism of Action: Blocks dopamine receptors as well as H1 receptors (antiemetic effects, sedation)

- Common Uses: Vertigo (chronic dizziness), nausea/vomiting, motion sickness
- Memorable Side Effects: Sedation, fall risk, orthostatic BP changes, EPS, metabolic syndrome

- Whenever you see an order for meclizine to treat dizziness, be sure to assess other medications (sleepers, psych meds, opioids, antihypertensives, etc.) to make sure they aren't causing/worsening dizziness
- Can be given as needed
- Blocks H1 receptors, so sedation will be a good possibility
- Anticholinergic effects, but probably not a major deal if used as needed/infrequently at low doses

Antiemetic, Serotonin receptor antagonist

Example: Ondansetron (Zofran), Alosetron (Lotronex), Granisetron (Sancuso), Palonosetron (Aloxi)

Mechanism of Action: Blocks serotonin at 5HT3 receptors – acts centrally in the chemoreceptor trigger zone

NAPLEX Nuggets:

- Common Uses: Nausea/vomiting
- Memorable Side Effects: Constipation, sedation, QTc prolongation is a risk (pretty rare unless on other drugs that can contribute to QTc prolongation, i.e. amiodarone etc.)
- Frequently used in patients undergoing chemotherapy (nausea/vomiting common with chemo)
- Can be used as needed or scheduled
- Can cause QTc prolongation especially when used in combo with other QTc prolonging agents
- Has serotonin activity, be on the lookout for other serotonergic medications (like SSRI's, tramadol etc.)

Antiepileptic - Miscellaneous

Example: Carbamazepine (Tegretol)

Mechanism of Action: Multiple mechanisms, including altering sodium ion flow across cell membranes

NAPLEX Nuggets:

- Common Uses: Seizures, trigeminal neuralgia, bipolar disorder
- Memorable Side Effects: sedation, dizziness, rash, hyponatremia (SIADH), N/V
- Enzyme inducer, CYP3A4 so can decrease concentrations of multiple other meds (lots of drug interactions)
- Can "auto-induce" its own metabolism
- Liver Function, CBC, and sodium are important monitoring parameters
- Lots of wacky side effects (rash, liver function, hyponatremia, CBC changes) with this medication
- Levels likely not necessary for patients using this med for trigeminal neuralgia unless signs of toxicity
- Sedation, confusion, falls are possible with toxicity
- 4-12 mcg/mL is considered "normal" therapeutic concentration for seizures

Antiepileptic, Analgesic, GABA Analog

Example: Gabapentin (Neurontin), Pregabalin (Lyrica)

Mechanism of Action: Not very clear, but may modulate excitatory neurotransmitters – structure related to GABA, but doesn't actually bind GABA

NAPLEX Nuggets:
- Common Uses: Neuropathy, various pain syndromes, seizures
- Memorable Side Effects: Sedation, dizziness, edema
- Generally classified as an anti-seizure medication, but most often used for neuropathy
- Keep an eye out for patients with kidney disease who may be experiencing side effects as they can accumulate in patients with poor renal function
- Watch out for dizziness and sedation in our elderly patients as this can potentially contribute to falls
- Weight gain in the form of edema may potentially happen; be on the lookout for patients with a history CHF and edema issues, as well as those who may already be receiving diuretics like furosemide
- Pregabalin in general has a very similar mechanism of action to gabapentin, so it may also potentially be used (more expensive at this time)
- As dose of gabapentin goes up, % absorbed goes down – giving pregabalin a potential advantage at higher doses

Antiepileptic, Anti-migraine, Miscellaneous

Example: Topiramate (Topamax)

Mechanism of Action: Not well understood; possible effects on sodium channels as well as GABA receptors

NAPLEX Nuggets:

- Common Uses: Seizures, migraines
- Memorable Side Effects: "Dopamax, Topamax" – can cause cognitive impairment, sedation
- Cognitive slowing is probably the most concerning adverse effect for patients
- With the indication of migraines being a common issue with women of child-bearing age, be sure to remember that topiramate can reduce the effects of estrogen containing birth control
- Used for migraine prophylaxis, NOT acute relief
- With any medication being used to treat seizures, it is very important to not abruptly stop a medication unless there is a very good reason (serious side effect etc.)
- Weight loss could potentially be a beneficial adverse effect in an overweight seizure or migraine patient

Antiepileptic, Miscellaneous

Example: Phenytoin (Dilantin)

Mechanism of Action: Has effects on sodium movement across cells – stabilizes the cell membrane

NAPLEX Nuggets:
- Common Uses: Seizures
- Memorable Side Effects: GI, CNS changes, ataxia, vitamin D deficiency, liver function changes (rare)
- Be on the lookout for drug interactions (a few examples: fluconazole, amiodarone, alcohol, cimetidine, fluvoxamine, etc.) – if new meds are started, I would recommend looking up potential interactions
- Narrow therapeutic window drug - Very sensitive to changes in dose (small increase may lead to toxicity)
- Michaelis-Menten kinetics
- Usual phenytoin level is from 10-20 (can be misleading if patient has low albumin), obtaining a free level is considered best, but not possible by all laboratories (target free level is generally 1-2)
- Toxicity similar to alcohol toxicity in many ways...ataxia (difficulty walking), confusion, GI side effects like nausea, slurred speech, etc.

Antiepileptic, Mood stabilizer - Miscellaneous

Example: Divalproex (Valproic Acid, Depakote)

Mechanism of Action: Increases GABA activity (inhibitory neurotransmitter), not very well understood

NAPLEX Nuggets:
- Common Uses: Seizures, bipolar disorder, migraine prophylaxis
- Memorable Side Effects: CNS (sedation, dizziness), GI (N/V/stomach pain), hair loss – lots of rare side effects: possible effects on platelets, ammonia levels, LFTs etc.
- Checking drug levels usually not as important when using for mood or headaches (compared to seizures) unless trying to rule out toxicity
- Frequent dosing - 2 or 3 times per day
- Critical to ensure patients are taking! (Especially for seizures)
- If using for seizures, be sure to have patient assess for meds that lower seizure threshold (bupropion, tramadol are classic examples)
- Does have some drug interactions (i.e. lamotrigine)
- Pregnancy category X for Migraines
- Usual target level for seizures is 50-100
- Acute mania in bipolar disorder, may try to push dose to level of 125 if necessary
- Be aware of multiple dosage forms, and that changes in dosage form can affect levels – may want to check levels following conversion (long acting, sprinkles, liquid etc.)

Antifungal, Azole

Example: Fluconazole (Diflucan), Voriconazole (Vfend), Itraconazole (Sporanox)

Mechanism of Action: Ultimately inhibits formation in fungal cell membrane

NAPLEX Nuggets:
- Common Uses: Fungal infections like candidiasis, Cryptococcus, Aspergillus
- Memorable Side Effects: GI side effects most common, Liver failure (very rare) more likely with chronic use
- Classically used to treat yeast infections (Candidiasis) and many simple patients may only require one dose (fluconazole)
- Notorious cause of drug interactions via CYP 3A4 inhibition – It can increase concentrations of statins, seizure medications, and many more! (if you see patients started on this medication, be sure to look up possible drug interactions)
- Fungal infections are much more common in patients who are immunocompromised (i.e. AIDS, patient on immunosuppressant medications, etc.)
- Can potentially cause prolonged QTc intervals especially in patients on other medications that prolong the QTc

Antigout - Miscellaneous

Example: Colchicine (Colcrys)

Mechanism of Action: Inhibits Beta-tubulin ultimately inhibiting action of neutrophils that may contribute to gout symptoms

NAPLEX Nuggets:
- Common Uses: Gout flare or prophylaxis
- Memorable Side Effects: Diarrhea, nausea
- Diarrhea very prominent side effect (up to half of patients)
- Cleared by the kidney, so may need to use lower doses in CKD
- Can be used for acute gout flare or prophylaxis (unique from allopurinol which is only used for prophylaxis of gout)
- Always be on the lookout for medications that can elevate uric acid when you see an Rx for colchicine like thiazide diuretics, niacin etc.

Antihistamines – 2nd Generation

Example: Cetirizine (Zyrtec), Loratadine (Claritin), Fexofenadine (Allegra)

Mechanism of Action: Blocks H1 receptors preventing the activity of histamine

NAPLEX Nuggets:
- Common Uses: Allergic rhinitis, itching
- Memorable Side Effects: Sedation (much less than 1st generation antihistamines like diphenhydramine or hydroxyzine), mildly anticholinergic
- Second generation H1 blockers are generally first line for seasonal allergies as they are more tolerable than first generation antihistamines
- Generally less sedating and less anticholinergic effects than first generation
- Remember that histamine 1 receptor blockers are generally called antihistamines, while histamine 2 receptor blockers are acid blockers used for GI issues (ranitidine, famotidine, etc.)
- Often with antihistamines, if one doesn't work, patients may try another one from the same class
- Can be used in combinations with pseudoephedrine (i.e. Zyrtec - D, Claritin – D)

Antihypertensive, Alpha-2 agonist

Example: Clonidine (Catapres), Guanfacine (Tenex), Methyldopa (Aldomet)

Mechanism of Action: Centrally acting alpha-2 agonist which results in decreased sympathetic activity and drop in blood pressure

NAPLEX Nuggets:

- Common Uses: Hypertension, psych issues like ADHD, opioid withdrawal symptoms (clonidine)
- Memorable Side Effects: Drowsiness, dizziness, dry mouth
- Not the best in the elderly (on Beer's list)
- Mainly used in hypertension, but occasionally will see it used off label for various psych issues
- Clonidine comes in a patch formulation (and oral tabs) which may be advantageous for patients who can't swallow, take pills, etc.
- Low BP and Pulse is possible
- Sedating which can be a significant problem especially in the elderly
- Methyldopa (Labetalol, nifedipine) considered one of the drugs of choice for hypertension in pregnancy

Antihypertensive, Angiotensin Receptor Blocker (ARB)

Example: Irbesartan (Avapro), Candesartan (Atacand), Losartan (Cozaar), Olmesartan (Benicar), Valsartan (Diovan), Telmisartan (Micardis)

Mechanism of Action: Blocks the angiotensin 2 receptor – ends up preventing vasoconstriction, aldosterone release etc. (remember aldosterone antagonists can raise potassium just like ARBs and ACE Inhibitors)

NAPLEX Nuggets:
- Common Uses: hypertension, heart failure
- Memorable Side Effects: hyperkalemia, exacerbate/worsen kidney function, low blood pressure
- When you think of ARBs and ACE inhibitors, you can lump the side effects together as they are overall the same
- One major exception to the above rule is the side effect of cough; cough usually doesn't happen with ARBs, and you will see patients who develop cough on an ACE inhibitor be transitioned to an ARB
- Kidney function changes and monitoring of potassium is critical when doses are changed or an ARB is initiated
- This worsening kidney function risk increases in patients who may be taking NSAIDs and/or diuretics
- As with any medication used to treat hypertension, we need to educate our patients to rise slowly when getting up to minimize risk of orthostatic (sometimes called postural) hypotension

Antihypertensive, Antianginal, Nitrate

Example: Nitroglycerine (Nitrostat), Isosorbide Dinitrate (Isordil), Isosorbide Mononitrate (Imdur)

Mechanism of Action: Metabolized into nitric oxide which leads to smooth muscle relaxation (vasodilation)

NAPLEX Nuggets:
- Common Uses: angina (chest pain)
- Memorable Side Effects: Low BP, headache
- Sublingual used most commonly for acute relief of chest pain (angina)
- Make sure patients are well educated on chest pain that doesn't resolve with use (emergency)
- For immediate release nitroglycerine recommended to only use every 5 minutes as needed(max of 3 tabs)
- Longer acting products available dosed daily (isosorbide mononitrate) or multiple times daily (isosorbide dinitrate)
- Patch formulation available as well for those that have trouble swallowing or tolerating the oral formulation
- Development of tolerance possible with overuse

Antihypertensive, Potassium Sparing Diuretic, Aldosterone antagonist

Example: Spironolactone (Aldactone), Eplerenone (Inspra)

Mechanism of Action: Aldosterone antagonist – increases water excretion and sodium (diuretic) but spares potassium (can increase potassium levels)

NAPLEX Nuggets:
- Common Uses: Heart failure, cirrhosis with ascites
- Memorable Side Effects: hyperkalemia, gynecomastia, low BP, hyponatremia, dehydration
- Much like all diuretics, in relation to the effects on the kidney, the risk of overdiuresis (promoting too much fluid loss) is worsening kidney function by inadequate flow through the kidney
- The development of "moobs" (man boobs) and breast tenderness can be very troubling for male patients on spironolactone (gynecomastia)
- We can often reduce the potassium supplementation (especially patients on high doses of KCl supplements) burden by using potassium sparing diuretics

Antihypertensive, Thiazide Diuretic

Example: Hydrochlorothiazide (Hydrodiuril), Chlorthalidone (Thalitone), Chlorothiazide (Diuril)

Mechanism of Action: Inhibit sodium/chloride transporter in the distal tubules

NAPLEX Nuggets:
- Common Use: hypertension, edema, heart failure
- Memorable Side Effects: (similar to loop diuretics) they are going to increase urine output and decrease amount of volume in the body which can lead to frequent urination, electrolyte depletion, low blood pressure, and increased risk of kidney failure
- One of the major differences between loops and thiazides are that thiazides can INCREASE serum calcium while loops will reduce it
- While loop diuretics can potentially cause hyperuricemia (elevated uric acid possibly contributing to or exacerbating gout), thiazides are classically known to do this – Be on the lookout when gout medications are being added or patients are reporting gout flares
- Hydrochlorothiazide (HCTZ) is used in a ton of medication combinations for hypertension; Examples: Triamterene/HCTZ, Lisinopril/HCTZ etc. This can often confuse patients and they may not realize that they are actually receiving two medications
- Kidney function and electrolytes are going to be the primary labs to monitor – potassium supplementation is common in patients taking diuretics
- Watch the timing of diuretics – too close to evening can be very problematic as patients will be getting up to go to the bathroom all night
- May not be that effective with poor kidney function (CrCl <30)

Antihypertensive, Vasodilator

Example: Nitroprusside (Nitropress)

Mechanism of Action: Direct vasodilation on vessel smooth muscle

NAPLEX Nuggets:
- Common Uses: Hypertensive crisis, heart failure
- Memorable Side Effects: Low blood pressure, changes in heart rate, dizziness, metabolic acidosis
- Drops blood pressure – risk of too much drug is low blood pressure
- Injection type reaction can happen - pain, redness, rash, warmth
- Cyanide toxicity is a black box warning if used at too high of a dose or for too long

Antilipemic

Example: Niacin (Niaspan)

Mechanism of Action: Converted to nicotinamide which can affect lipid metabolism

NAPLEX Nuggets:
- Common Uses: Hyperlipidemia
- Memorable Side Effects: Flushing, GI, increase uric acid
- Flushing from niacin can be treated with aspirin
- Slow release formulation may help minimize flushing as well
- Can possibly exacerbate gout (increase uric acid)
- Possibly can increase blood sugars, but usually not clinically significant – if a patient had persistent high blood sugars, might be a good idea to avoid niacin
- Rare possibility of liver issues

Anti-migraine, Triptan

Example: Sumatriptan (Imitrex), Frovatriptan (Frova), Maxalt (Rizatriptan)

Mechanism of Action: Serotonin 5HT agonist – which causes vasoconstriction and reduction in inflammation associated with migraine

NAPLEX Nuggets:
- Common Uses: Acute relief of migraine
- Memorable Side Effects: Dizziness, changes in CNS
- Meant for acute relief of migraine, not prophylaxis
- Comes in multiple formulations (not just oral), injection, nasal, etc. as some may struggle with nausea when they have a migraine
- Be sure to assess frequent use, if using frequently, need to have control of migraines assessed and have controller medication added (valproic acid, propranolol, topiramate, etc.)
- Often used with NSAIDs (i.e. naproxen) in migraine treatment
- Does have serotonin activity so could potentially contribute to serotonin syndrome (higher risk in patients already on SSRI's, tramadol etc.)

Anti-Parkinson's – Dopamine Replacement

Example: Carbidopa/levodopa (Sinemet)

Mechanism of Action: Levodopa crosses the blood brain barrier and gets converted to dopamine; carbidopa prevents the peripheral breakdown of levodopa

NAPLEX Nuggets:
- Common Uses: Parkinson's, restless leg syndrome
- Memorable Side Effects: Nausea/vomiting, hallucinations, orthostasis
- Levodopa replaces the body's dopamine supply (shortage of dopamine in Parkinson's)
- Can cause psychotic type symptoms (remember that antipsychotics block dopamine)
- GI upset/nausea is common
- Frequent dosing (up to 6-8 times per day) may be necessary depending upon patient's symptoms
- May see used at night for RLS
- Dopamine blockers (i.e. antipsychotics, metoclopramide, etc.) can exacerbate or reduce efficacy of Sinemet

Anti-Parkinson's agent, Dopamine Agonist

Example: Pramipexole (Mirapex), Ropinirole (Requip)

Mechanism of Action: Stimulates dopamine receptors

NAPLEX Nuggets:

- Common Uses: Restless Legs Syndrome, Parkinson's disorder
- Memorable Side Effects: Orthostasis, edema, OCD symptoms (very rare)
- Indicated for Parkinson's but more commonly drug of choice for RLS
- Often patients struggle with RLS at night, so if you see it dosed once daily at night, this is likely the indication
- Keep an eye out for orthostasis, especially in the elderly and patients who may also be receiving numerous antihypertensives already
- Make sure the medication actually helps the patient, have often seen this added when diagnosis is unclear; cramps versus spasms, versus RLS
- Possible for iron deficiency to contribute or cause RLS symptoms

Antiplatelet, Thienopyridine

Example: Clopidogrel (Plavix), Prasugrel (Effient), Ticlopidine

Mechanism of Action: Blocks ADP receptors P2Y12 which leads to inhibition of platelets

NAPLEX Nuggets:
- Common Uses: MI, Stroke prevention
- Memorable Side Effects: Bleeding (GI, nose bleeds, bruising etc.)
- Often used after a heart attack (acute coronary syndrome) with aspirin to prevent further heart attacks; how long a patient should remain on this medication can vary depending upon cardiac and/or stroke risk – length of therapy should be addressed by the primary provider and in many situations may be 12 months, but can be longer or indefinite depending upon risk factors
- Clopidogrel is a common substitute if a patient cannot take or tolerate aspirin to help prevent stroke or heart attack
- Due to its ability to inhibit platelets, the major complication is bleeding – assess patients for bruising, blood in the stool, any abnormal sign of bleeding etc.
- CBC (hemoglobin and platelets in particular) are going to be one of the most important labs to monitor
- Ticlopidine is rarely used – boxed warning for hematologic toxicity, neutropenia etc.

Antitussive - Miscellaneous

Example: Benzonatate (Tessalon)

Mechanism of Action: Anesthetic effects on respiratory tract resulting in cough suppression

NAPLEX Nuggets:
- Memorable Side Effects: Usually pretty well tolerated, GI/possible CNS effects (rare)
- Very important to identify why patient is coughing
- If coughing has been going on a long time be sure patients get assessed
- ACE Inhibitors are classic cause of drug induced cough
- An atypical cause of cough that won't resolve is heartburn or GERD (especially in elderly or young)
- Asthma is another potential cause of chronic cough

Antiviral

Example: Acyclovir (Zovirax), Valacyclovir (Valtrex)

Mechanism of Action: Inhibits DNA synthesis and viral replication

NAPLEX Nuggets:
- Typically for most viral infections, the sooner treatment is started once an infection is identified, the better
- You can think of acyclovir and valacyclovir as essentially the same...the big advantage of valacyclovir is that patients don't need to take it so many times per day (acyclovir may need to be dosed up to 5 times per day which is far from ideal for our patients)
- Common Uses: Shingles, genital herpes, chicken pox
- Monitor for GI side effects, and Liver Function Tests will be more important if long term use is necessary
- May need to reduce dose and/or have a heightened awareness for potential adverse effects in patients with poor kidney function
- CNS toxicity possible (risk especially with high doses/accumulating drug in CKD)
- Also comes in a topical form that can be used for cold sores (herpes labialis) or Genital Herpes Simplex Virus

Antiviral, Neuraminidase Inhibitor

Example: Oseltamivir (Tamiflu), Zanamivir (Relenza)

Mechanism of Action: Inhibits viral neuraminidase, preventing influenza virus from replicating

NAPLEX Nuggets:
- Common Uses: Influenza treatment and prophylaxis
- Memorable Side Effects: GI, psych events like delirium (rare, more likely in pediatrics)
- Oseltamivir is drug of choice for influenza prophylaxis or treatment
- Prophylaxis is especially common for patients at high risk who've been exposed to infected individuals (immunosuppressed, elderly, healthcare institution – i.e. nursing home)
- Dose adjustments in patients with poor kidney function (oseltamivir)
- GI upset is going to be the most common side effect (oseltamivir)
- With or without food is ok, but likely better tolerated by the stomach with food (oseltamivir)
- Encourage influenza vaccination!
- Zanamivir available as inhalation product but seldom used

Anxiolytics - Miscellaneous

Example: Buspirone (Buspar)

Mechanism of Action: Not well known, possible effects on serotonin, dopamine

NAPLEX Nuggets:

- Memorable Side Effects: Sedation (pretty well tolerated in the elderly compared to other anti-anxiety medications)
- Usually a much safer choice for treatment of anxiety versus benzodiazepines (especially elderly)
- Big disadvantage is they take a while (weeks to months) to show benefit for anxiety compared to benzo's which work quickly for anxiety
- They don't work on an as needed basis
- Advantage versus benzodiazepines - Not a controlled substance in the U.S.
- Disadvantage - Usually dosed multiple times per day

Barbituates

Example: Phenobarbital

Mechanism of Action: Depress the CNS, not well understood

NAPLEX Nuggets:
- Old antiseizure medication rarely used due to adverse effects
- Also has enzyme inducing activity and has lots of drug interactions
- May decrease Vitamin D levels
- Primidone is a prodrug that gets metabolized to phenobarbital
- Many similar side effects to alcohol (sedation, fall risk, confusion etc.)

Benzodiazepines

Example: Alprazolam (Xanax), Lorazepam (Ativan), Diazepam (Valium), Temazepam (Restoril), Midazolam (Versed), Oxazepam (Serax), Clonazepam (Klonopin)

Mechanism of Action: enhances activity of GABA (an inhibitor neurotransmitter that causes sedation)

NAPLEX Nuggets:
- Common Uses: Anxiety, insomnia, sedation, seizures
- Memorable Side Effects: sedation, confusion, fall risk, dizziness
- The best way I remember benzodiazepines is that they are very close to "alcohol in a pill"
- Sedation, slurred speech, confusion, trouble walking (ataxia) etc. are all common with benzo's/alcohol; they are also commonly used in alcohol withdrawal protocols
- Be cautious with patients on higher doses of benzodiazepines to make sure they aren't abruptly stopped (risk of withdrawal)
- Educate patients on driving/operating machinery (remember that benzodiazepines are often used for sleep as well as anxiety)
- Flumazenil is antidote in overdose
- Unlike SSRI's for anxiety, a great advantage of benzo's are that they work quickly and can be used as needed
- Falls in the elderly is a big downside to using these medications
- Benzo's are a controlled substance, i.e. they can cause addiction, etc.
- Midazolam only used in the hospital setting for its sedative properties in anesthesia for various procedures/surgery
- Remember "LOT", lorazepam, oxazepam, temazepam – generally considered safer in the elderly due to the way

they are metabolized (the drugs don't hang around in the body)

- Diazepam has a rectal formulation for seizures

Beta-Blockers (Systemic)

Example: Metoprolol (Lopressor or Toprol), Atenolol (Tenormin), Labetalol (Trandate), Carvedilol (Coreg), Bisoprolol (Zebeta), Esmolol (Brevibloc), Nebivolol (Bystolic), Propranolol (Inderal), Nadolol (Corgard), Sotalol (Betapace)

Mechanism of Action: Blocks beta receptors primarily causing drop in pulse and blood pressure

NAPLEX Nuggets:
- Common Uses: Hypertension, Afib
- Trick to remembering beta receptors: You have 1 heart and 2 lungs (beta-1 is primarily on the heart and beta-2 primarily in the lungs). You will see beta receptors again with respiratory medications. If beta-1 is stimulated, heart rate increases. If beta-1 is blocked, heart rate decreases.
- Atenolol, metoprolol, Bisoprolol, Esmolol, Nebivolol are considered relatively selective for beta-1 only
- Normal pulse ranges from 60-100, be cautious about starting or further increasing a beta blocker if patients pulse is already around that 60 mark or less
- Propranolol and Nadolol are non-selective
- Non-selective beta blockers run a higher risk of masking hypoglycemia and are more likely to block effects of beta agonists like albuterol (problematic especially in asthma/respiratory diseases)
- Non-selective agents (propranolol) are often utilized in migraines, portal hypertension (cirrhosis patients), and essential tremor
- Carvedilol, Labetalol have alpha blocking activity
- Common compelling indications for beta-blockers; CHF, Angina, Post-MI
- Sotalol is considered an antiarrhythmic that has Class 2, 3, and beta-blocking effects

Bisphosphonates

Example: Alendronate (Fosamax), Risedronate (Actonel), Ibandronate (Boniva), Zoledronic acid (Reclast)

Mechanism of Action: Inhibits osteoclasts (osteoclasts break down bone)

NAPLEX Nuggets:
- Memorable Side Effects: Esophageal ulceration (administration procedure important to decrease this risk), GI side effects in general (with oral products)
- Timing of administration is critical for oral bisphosphonates! Take on an empty stomach, usually right away in the morning with 6-8 ounces of plain water 30 minutes prior to any food or drink (that isn't plain water)
- Have patient remain sitting or standing upright for 30 minutes (this is to reduce the risk of esophageal irritation or ulceration)
- Absorption will be limited and drug will not be effective if taken with food or other medications
- After 3-5 years of bisphosphonate use, some lower risk patients may be able to have the medication reassessed for ongoing need
- Osteonecrosis (destruction or dying) of the jaw is extremely rare; patients may be at increased risk if recently had an invasive dental procedure
- Be cautious with oral bisphosphonates in patients who already have esophageal or GI related concerns (GI bleed or ulcer history)
- Always important to assess adequate vitamin D and calcium intake
- Zoledronic acid is administered once yearly for osteoporosis and can also be used to treat hypercalcemia of malignancy (Not recommended for patients with CrCl <35)

- Ibandronate (oral) is given once month (a nice advantage if patients don't like weekly administration of commonly used alendronate)

Calcium Channel Blocker (non-dihydropyridine), antiarrhythmic

Example: Diltiazem (Cardizem CD, Cartia XT), Verapamil (Verelan)

Mechanism of Action: Blocks calcium channels resulting in vasodilation and cardiac relaxation

NAPLEX Nuggets:
- Common Uses: Atrial fibrillation, hypertension
- Used for rate control (not rhythm) in AFib
- Memorable Side Effects: Low pulse, low BP, constipation, edema
- Very important distinction: Verapamil and Diltiazem (non-dihydropyridine's) are the calcium channel blockers that act on the heart AND blood vessels; you will not see amlodipine and nifedipine used in atrial fibrillation, because their activity is primarily on the vessels. This also means that pulse monitoring will not be necessary with nifedipine and amlodipine
- The higher you push the dose on these medications, the more likely you will see the side effect of edema; keep an eye out for new diuretic Rx's to treat the edema caused by the calcium channel blockers
- CYP3A4 interaction potential
- Simvastatin is a very common medication that interacts with diltiazem
- Diltiazem comes in several different formulations (long acting, short acting etc.), make sure you have the right one

Calcium Channel Blockers - Dihydropyridine

Example: Amlodipine (Norvasc), Felodipine (Plendil), Nifedipine (Nifedical)

Mechanism of Action: blocks calcium ions from entering voltage smooth muscle, resulting in relaxation (vasodilation) – dihydropyridine calcium channel blocker

NAPLEX Nuggets:
- Very important distinction: You will not see amlodipine used in atrial fibrillation, because its activity is primarily on the vessels; this differs from non-dihydropyridine calcium channel blockers like verapamil and diltiazem that act on the heart AND blood vessels; This also means that pulse monitoring will not be normally necessary with dihydropyridines
- Commonly used for hypertension
- The higher you push the dose on these medications, the more likely you will see the side effect of edema
- Constipation is another common side effect with CCB's
- Keep an eye out for new requirement of diuretic Rx's to treat the edema caused by the calcium channel blockers
- Educate our patients to get up slowly to minimize risk of orthostatic hypotension
- Amlodipine is usually only dosed once daily which is nice, but you may see it twice daily if the provider feels blood pressure increases as the effects are wearing off
- Simvastatin is a very common medication that interacts with "most" of the calcium channel blockers, including amlodipine

Carbapenem Antibiotics

Example: Ertapenem (Invanz), Imipenem/Cilastatin (Primaxin), Meropenem (Merrem), Doripenem (Doribax)

Mechanism of Action: Bind at the penicillin binding proteins on bacterial cell walls and disrupts formation thus inhibiting growth

NAPLEX Nuggets:
- Very broad spectrum antibiotics (reserved for very bad/resistant infections)
- Ertapenem not quite as broad and doesn't work well for Pseudomonas
- Rarely associated with seizures
- Bigger guns being used, risk for CDiff especially with prolonged treatment
- May decrease valproic acid concentrations (very careful if using for seizures)
- Cilastatin prevents kidneys from eliminating imipenem

Central Nervous System (CNS) - Stimulants

Example: Amphetamine/Dextroamphetamine (Adderall), Methylphenidate (Ritalin), Dexmethylphenidate (Focalin), Lisdexamfetamine (Vyvanse)

Mechanism of Action: Stimulates release of norepinephrine and dopamine leading to CNS stimulation

NAPLEX Nuggets:
- Common Uses: ADHD
- Remembering that this medication ramps you up (stimulant) will help you remember its side effects (anxiety, insomnia, weight loss, poor appetite, increased BP, increased pulse etc.)
- Timing of dosing can be important to avoid insomnia and maximize benefit
- When used in pediatrics, poor appetite can be a significant problem and should be something that should be assessed
- BP and Pulse monitoring is important
- Be cautious in adult patients who may already be at cardiovascular risk (hypertension, etc.)
- Schedule 2 controlled substance, addictive

Cephalosporin – Fifth Generation

Example: Ceftaroline (Teflaro)

Mechanism of Action: Inhibits bacterial cell wall formation

NAPLEX Nuggets:
- MRSA activity
- Heightened effect versus Strep Pneumonia as well

Cephalosporin – Fourth Generation

Example: Cefepime (Maxipime)

Mechanism of Action: Inhibits bacterial cell wall formation

NAPLEX Nuggets:
- Big advantage is coverage against pseudomonas

Cephalosporin – Second Generation

Example: Cefaclor (Ceclor), Cefotetan, Cefoxitin (Mefoxin), Cefprozil, Cefuoxime (Ceftin)

Mechanism of Action: Inhibits bacterial cell wall formation

NAPLEX Nuggets:

- Common Uses: surgical prophylaxis, endocarditis (if bacteria sensitive), skin infections
- Memorable Side Effects: GI side effects most common, allergy, rash
- Alternative to penicillin antibiotics (very low risk of cross reactivity, but is possible), can be used in pediatrics as alternative for bacterial URI or ear infection
- If using for treatment of an active infection, patients should begin improving within a couple days if drug is working
- Gram positive bacteria is primary coverage
- Minimal activity against MRSA
- Possible option in pregnancy for UTI (category B) but most UTI's are caused by gram negative so coverage may not be very good

Cephalosporin – Third Generation

Example: Cefdinir, Cefotaxime (Claforan), Ceftazidime (Fortaz), Ceftriaxone (Rocephin)

Mechanism of Action: Inhibits bacterial cell wall formation

NAPLEX Nuggets:
- Common Uses: Significantly more gram negative coverage than 1st and 2nd generation, cephalosporins, used frequently in pneumonia (ceftriaxone), Pseudomonas activity (ceftazidime), meningitis, endocarditis
- Memorable Side Effects: GI side effects most common (for oral meds), allergy, rash
- Minimal activity against MRSA
- Ceftriaxone injection (I.M.) co-administered with lidocaine to minimize pain
- Ceftriaxone used for gonorrhea

Cephalosporin First Generation

Example: Cefadroxil, Cefazolin, Cephalexin (Keflex)

Mechanism of Action: Inhibits bacterial cell wall formation

NAPLEX Nuggets:

- Common Uses: surgical prophylaxis, endocarditis (if bacteria sensitive), skin infections
- Memorable Side Effects: GI side effects most common, allergy, rash
- Often used in surgery prophylaxis to prevent infections (cefazolin)
- Alternative to penicillin antibiotics (low risk of cross reactivity, but is possible)
- If using for treatment of an active infection, patients should begin improving within a couple days if drug is working
- Gram positive bacteria is primary coverage
- Minimal activity against MRSA
- Possible option in pregnancy for UTI (category B) but most UTI's are caused by gram negative so coverage may not be very good

Colony Stimulating Factor (CSF) Agents, Antineutropenia Agents

Example: Filgrastim (Neupogen), Pegfilgrastim (Neulasta)

Mechanism of Action: Stimulates production of WBC's (neutrophils primarily)

NAPLEX Nuggets:
- Common Uses: Prevention of neutropenia in chemo patients
- Memorable Side Effects: Ostealgia (bone pain), anaphylaxis (rare)
- Helps patients continue on chemotherapy by increasing white blood cells
- Bone pain is common (remember that it stimulates bone marrow which resides inside the bones – source of pain)
- CBC (white blood cell count is incredibly important to monitor for response to treatment)
- Fever and signs of infection are also incredibly important to watch for in a patient on CSF – remember that we are treating neutropenia so patient are at risk of infection
- Long acting version of filgrastim = pegfilgrastim (dosed less frequently is advantage, but more $)
- Acetaminophen or NSAIDs commonly used to help with bone pain

COMT Inhibitors

Example: Entacapone (Comtan), Tolcapone (Tasmar)

Mechanism of Action: Inhibits catechol-O-methyltransferase which prevents the breakdown of levodopa and therefore enhances its activity

NAPLEX Nuggets:
- Always give with Sinemet (levodopa)
- Tolcapone is rarely used due to hepatotoxicity
- Adverse effect profile will likely be mostly due to an increase in levodopa (i.e. hallucinations, GI, etc.)

Cox-2 Inhibtors

Example: Celecoxib (Celebrex)

Mechanism of Action: Inhibits Cyclooxygenase-2 preferentially (COX-2); results in a reduction in prostaglandins which cause pain, fever, inflammation

NAPLEX Nuggets:
- Common Uses: Pain, inflammation, rheumatoid arthritis
- Memorable Side Effects: GI ulcer (less than traditional NSAIDs), worsening kidney function, edema, hypertension
- COX-2 inhibitors can cause GI bleed, but the risk is much less than traditional NSAIDs - risk increases in the elderly and those on medications that increase risk of bleeding (anticoagulants and antiplatelet medications)
- COX-2 inhibitors can contribute to edema and exacerbate CHF (congestive heart failure); be on the lookout and have celecoxib reassessed if you see a patient with a CHF exacerbation or a patient requiring increasing diuretics like furosemide
- Celecoxib can cause worsening kidney function (creatinine should be monitored); this risk can be greatly increased in patients on ACE Inhibitors or ARBs and/or diuretic type medications
- When you think of celecoxib, think NSAID side effects with less GI risk
- Boxed warning for increased risk of heart attack (MI) and stroke

Decongestant

Example: Pseudoephedrine (Sudafed)

Mechanism of Action: Stimulates alpha receptors causing vasoconstriction (beneficial in the respiratory tract)

NAPLEX Nuggets:
- Common Uses: Nasal congestion
- Memorable Side Effects: hypertension, urinary retention (watch out for BPH patients), dry mouth, anxiety
- Watch out for elderly/patients at high risk for cardiovascular problems as it can raise BP
- Can exacerbate BPH
- Can cause/worsen insomnia and/or anxiety
- Use is restricted in the U.S. – need to sign a log book to obtain it from the pharmacist; component necessary for making methamphetamine

DMARD (antirheumatic), TNF blocker

Example: Etanercept (Enbrel), Adalimumab (Humira), Infliximab (Remicade)

Mechanism of Action: Blocks tumor necrosis factor (TNF) – TNF plays a role in the inflammatory process

NAPLEX Nuggets:

- Common Uses: rheumatoid arthritis, psoriasis/psoriatic arthritis, ulcerative colitis, Crohn's disease
- Memorable Side Effects: Infection and malignancy risk (suppresses immune system), injection site reaction
- May see pretreatment with analgesics, H1 blockers or even corticosteroids to minimize/prevent injection site reaction
- Watch for frequent or serious infections (suppresses immune system)
- Acts as a controller of inflammatory conditions, not immediate relief
- Expensive!!!
- Refrigerated; but may warm to room temp to make injection less painful

DMARD (Disease modifying antirheumatic drug)

Example: Methotrexate (Rheumatrex), Sulfasalazine (Azulfidine), Hydroxychloroquine (Plaquenil)

Mechanism of Action: Not very well understood for treatment of inflammatory/immune disease, but thought to impair immune function leading to benefit

NAPLEX Nuggets:
- Common Uses: Rheumatoid arthritis, psoriasis, Crohn's, Ulcerative Colitis, certain cancers - methotrexate (much higher doses used in cancer treatment)
- Memorable Side Effects: Low WBC or platelet count, increased liver enzymes, GI (sulfasalazine)
- Oral DMARDs are first line for rheumatoid arthritis
- Usually dosed once weekly (methotrexate)
- Need to supplement folic acid when using chronically (methotrexate)
- May take weeks for a response, so likely will not be beneficial in acute flare of inflammation (NSAIDs or prednisone typically used for acute RA flare)
- Suppresses immune system so WBC and infection monitoring is important
- LFT's should also be monitored
- Hydroxychloroquine requires routine eye exams

Erythropoiesis Stimulating Agent (ESA)

Example: Darbepoetin alfa (Aranesp), Epoetin alfa (Epogen, Procrit)

Mechanism of Action: Stimulates the production of red blood cells (mimics the body's natural erythropoietin which is produced by the kidney)

NAPLEX Nuggets:
- Common Uses: Anemia from CKD, anemia from chemotherapy/cancer
- Memorable Side Effects: Hypertension, GI, Injection site reaction, increase clot risk (boxed warning)
- Lack of iron stores may inhibit response
- Monitor hemoglobin/hematocrit for response (should increase)
- Risk of hypertension
- There should be hold parameters in place (i.e. hold if hemoglobin is greater than 11)
- Darbepoetin alfa is the longer acting form of erythropoietin (advantage is you don't have to give it as often)
- Important boxed warning on increased risk of MI, stroke, blood clots

Estrogen and Progestin (Contraceptive)

Example: Ethinyl Estradiol and Norgestimate (Ortho-Cyclen, Sprintec, Ortho Tri-Cyclen Lo etc.)

Mechanism of Action: Inhibits ovulation by changing gonadotropin, FSH, and luteinizing hormone release

NAPLEX Nuggets:

- Common Uses: Contraception, Acne
- Memorable Side Effects: Abnormal vaginal bleeding, DVT, hypertension
- Age, Smoking can put patients at higher risk of clot
- Can exacerbate hypertension
- Adherence to regimen is very important to prevent unplanned pregnancy
- Enzyme inducers like carbamazepine, phenytoin can possibly reduce effectiveness of birth control
- Remember to advise backup protection if regimen is interrupted (one missed dose is ok as long as 2 tablets are taken the next day)
- 2 missed doses, take 2 tabs each of the next two days and continue schedule (backup contraception methods recommended)
- 3 or more, will have to start a new pack

Estrogen Replacement

Example: Conjugated Estrogen (Premarin)

Mechanism of Action: Mimics body's natural estrogen

NAPLEX Nuggets:
- Common Uses: Menopausal symptoms, osteoporosis, uterine bleeding, vaginal atrophy (due to menopause)
- Memorable Side Effects: GI side effects, clot formation (DVT/PE), increased risk of certain types of cancers
- Most often used for estrogen replacement in postmenopausal women
- Alleviates troublesome hot flashes
- Big risk is increase in certain types of cancer (endometrial, breast) as well as clot formation (DVT); long term use is not recommended if possible
- Positive bone effects (good in patients with osteoporosis, but seldom used for OP given risks mentioned above)

Expectorant

Example: Guaifenesin (Mucinex)

Mechanism of Action: Possibly increases amount of liquid in respiratory tract thereby has an expectorant effect

NAPLEX Nuggets:
- Common Uses: Promote loosening of mucus
- Memorable Side Effects: Pretty well tolerated overall
- Some argue that guaifenesin is not an effective expectorant
- Found in a ton of OTC cough and cold preparations
- There is an immediate release and extended release product
- Always important with over the counter medications to educate patients on factors that may help guide them on when to seek medical attention with common cold symptoms (symptoms greater than 7 days, continually worsening symptoms, significant fever, rash, underlying respiratory condition, high risk for complications etc.)

Folic Acid Supplement

Example: Folic Acid

Mechanism of Action: Replacement of dietary folic acid

NAPLEX Nuggets:
- Common Uses: Pregnancy, patients on methotrexate or other meds that cause low folic acid levels, folic acid deficiency
- Memorable Side Effects: GI upset if anything, but virtually no side effects, water soluble so won't accumulate
- Folic acid supplementation is recommended in pregnancy to minimize risk of neural tube defects
- Deficiency (B12 also) can lead to megaloblastic anemia (indicated by high MCV)
- Found in nearly all multivitamins
- Sulfasalazine and Trimethoprim are two medications that can potentially cause folic acid deficiency
- May need to replace folic acid in alcoholism
- Use with methotrexate also recommended

GLP-1 Agonists

Example: Exenatide (Byetta), Liraglutide (Victoza)

Mechanism of Action: Glucagon-like peptide-1 promotes a feeling of fullness and decreases food intake – these drugs are analogs of this endogenous hormone

NAPLEX Nuggets:
- GI is the major side effect (maybe that's why it causes weight loss?) – can be a really good thing in overweight type 2 diabetes patients
- Indicated for diabetes and/or weight loss
- Injection only is a downside
- Exenatide is twice daily vs. liraglutide once daily
- Expensive
- Long acting Exenatide available

Histamine Antagonist (H2 Receptor Blocker)

Example: Ranitidine (Zantac), Famotidine (Pepcid), Cimetidine (Tagamet), Nizatidine (Axid)

Mechanism of Action: Blocks histamine 2 receptors (H2 blocker) which results in reduced gastric acid secretion and a higher pH in the stomach

NAPLEX Nuggets:
- Uses: GERD, heartburn, GI bleed
- Memorable Side Effects: Pretty well tolerated overall (watch out for CNS changes in elderly and/or patients with poor kidney function)
- H2 blockers are cleared by the kidney, so they can accumulate/require dose adjustments in CKD
- Generally less effective at suppressing stomach acid than PPI's, but possibly slightly safer (less risk of osteoporosis, C. Diff etc. risk)
- Available over the counter, inexpensive
- CNS side effects likely more common in elderly, on higher doses, and in patients with kidney disease
- Generally used before PPI's if something more than Tums (calcium carbonate) is needed in pregnancy
- Cimetidine is notorious for CYP3A4 drug interactions

Hypnotics – "Z-drugs

Example: Zolpidem (Ambien), Eszopiclone (Lunesta), Zaleplon (Sonata)

Mechanism of Action: enhances activity of GABA (an inhibitor neurotransmitter that causes sedation)

NAPLEX Nuggets:
- Common Uses: Insomnia
- Memorable Side Effects: sedation, confusion, fall risk, dizziness, abnormal sleep behaviors (sleep walking, eating etc.)
- Similar side effect profile to benzodiazepines
- Often termed as a "Z" drug because they have a "z" in their name
- Be mindful of the morning after and make sure patients realize that driving and/or operating machinery can be extremely dangerous
- It is recommended to try to use these medications only for short term if possible
- Non-drug interventions such as sleep hygiene are the preferred treatment for insomnia
- Before this type of medication is prescribed, keep an eye out for patients who may be on stimulating type medications or medications that can contribute to insomnia and make sure that these are assessed prior to giving a sleep medication – classic examples: methylphenidate, prednisone, too much levothyroxine, etc.
- Schedule 4 controlled substance in the U.S.; there is a risk of addiction/dependence
- Can increase risk of falls in our elderly patients
- Similar mechanism to benzodiazepines

Hypoglycemia Antidote

Example: Glucagon (GlucaGen)

Mechanism of Action: Stimulates adenylate cyclase which results in increased glucose production causing an increase in blood sugar

NAPLEX Nuggets:

- Mechanism of Action: Common Uses: Treatment of hypoglycemia
- Memorable Side Effects: Hyperglycemia, change in BP/Pulse, GI
- Be sure caregivers are educated on how/when to use glucagon
- If alert without any mental status change, in most cases should be able to oral glucose vs. glucagon
- Risk of aspiration exists if try to give oral glucose gel (or other source of sugar) to a patient who is in and out of consciousness – so give glucagon in this case
- Close monitoring of blood glucose is obviously important
- IV Dextrose used if glucagon fails

Inhaled Anticholinergic

Example: Tiotropium (Spiriva), Aclidinium (Tudorza)

Mechanism of Action: Inhaled anticholinergic can open up airways and decrease secretions

NAPLEX Nuggets:
- Common Uses: COPD
- Memorable Side Effects: Dry mouth, cough, irritation to the lungs (usually pretty well tolerated) usually not clinically significant systemic absorption
- Primarily used for COPD, and because it has anticholinergic activity, it can help dry up the airways as well as open them up to allow for better breathing in patients who have think mucous/sputum
- It is long acting and meant to be used as a controller medication
- It will not provide acute relief from respiratory distress, not meant to be a rescue inhalation product
- Often by using this medication in COPD, our goal is likely to improve respiratory status, but also to reduce the amount of as needed albuterol and/or albuterol/ipratropium (Duoneb or Combivent)
- Tiotropium comes with a special delivery device and capsules; to prepare the device for use, the capsules are inserted into the device and punctured for the contents to be inhaled by the patient
- With the delivery device, it is imperative to assess if patients are able to adequately coordinate how to use the device as well as if they are able to inhale quickly and forcefully enough to get the drug into their lungs
- Systemic anticholinergic effects (can't spit, see, pee or poop) are usually not a concern as systemic absorption is low

Inhaled Corticosteroids

Example: Beclomethasone (Qvar), Budesonide (Pulmicort), Fluticasone (Flovent), Mometasone (Asmanex)

Mechanism of Action: Multiple suspected mechanisms, but end result is a decrease in inflammation in the respiratory tract

NAPLEX Nuggets:
- Very important to rinse following use to reduce the risk of thrush
- Not meant for acute respiratory distress/asthma attack
- Combo products available (steroid plus long acting beta agonist, i.e. Advair, Symbicort etc.)
- First line controller medication for asthma
- May help decrease exacerbations in COPD
- Systemic steroid adverse effects considered minimal to non-existent
- Budesonide available as nebulized formulation (good for pediatrics and geriatrics)

Insulin - Rapid Acting

Example: Aspart (Novolog), Glulisine (Apidra), Lispro (Humalog)

Mechanism of Action: Rapid acting insulin binds insulin receptor and causes reduction in blood glucose

NAPLEX Nuggets:

- Common Uses: diabetes, hyperkalemia
- Memorable Side Effects: Weight gain, hypoglycemia, injection site issues (rotating sites usually alleviates this problem)
- Rapid acting insulin – so you will see this used to quickly bring down blood sugar, compared to the long acting insulins like detemir and glargine
- Sliding scale insulin is not ideal for diabetes management as you often end up "chasing" blood sugars
- When giving rapid acting insulin, remember to be aware of hypoglycemia protocols (juice, glucose gel, saltine crackers etc., or glucagon if patient is incapable of taking oral food/liquid)
- In many type 2 diabetes patients uncontrolled by oral medications, a combination of long acting once daily with rapid acting insulin with meal(s) is often used
- With insulin products, some providers will use hold orders on rapid acting insulin if blood sugars are below a certain value (i.e. 100 mg/dL)
- Keep an eye out for patients who have a change in appetite as they may require a reduction or increase in insulin based upon their dietary intake
- Can be used in an acute hyperkalemia situation

Insulin Long Acting

Example: Insulin Glargine (Lantus), Insulin Detemir (Levemir)

Mechanism of Action: Long acting insulin causes reduction in blood glucose

NAPLEX Nuggets:
- Common Uses: Diabetes
- Memorable Side Effects: Weight gain, hypoglycemia, injection site issues (rotating sites usually alleviates this problem)
- Sometimes called "peakless" or "basal" insulin
- The intent with long acting insulin is to mimic the consistent low level output of insulin by the pancreas
- Usually dosed once daily, but providers may be more likely to try to do twice daily as the dose increases (more injections for the patient is the downside)
- Basal insulin in Type 2 diabetes is often (but doesn't have to be) used after patients have tried oral medications without successful decrease in A1C
- Hypoglycemia is always a concern with any insulin product

Iron Replacement

Example: Ferrous Sulfate (Slow Fe, FeroSul), Ferrous Gluconate (Fergon), Ferrous Fumurate (Ferretts), Polysaccharide Iron Complex (Ferrex, Niferex), Iron Sucrose (Venofer)

Mechanism of Action: Replaces body's iron stores

NAPLEX Nuggets:
- Common Uses: Iron deficiency anemia
- Memorable Side Effects: Constipation, black stools, GI pain
- Iron deficiency anemia is the most common use for iron supplements
- In patients with CKD, anemia may likely be due to kidney disease versus iron deficiency (erythropoietin is produced in the kidney)
- Constipation and black stools can be troublesome for patients – key education point as patients may use OTC laxatives if iron supplementation is necessary
- May be given with vitamin C to increase absorption (sometimes have seen with orange juice)
- Pearls for IV Iron Sucrose (Venofer)
  - Risk of anaphylaxis from infusion is a significant risk
  - Ferritin and hemoglobin are important labs to monitor
  - May cause hypotension (BP monitoring important)
- Ferrous Sulfate contains about 20% elemental iron (of 325 mg tab, 65 mg is elemental)
- Ferrous Fumarate is approximately 33% elemental iron
- Ferrous Gluconate is approximately 12% elemental iron

Laxative, Osmotic

Example: Polyethylene Glycol (Miralax), Milk of Magnesia (MOM), Lactulose (Enulose)

Mechanism of Action: Draws fluid into the GI tract stimulating peristalsis (GI muscles activating to produce bowel movement)

NAPLEX Nuggets:
- Common Uses: Constipation, reduce ammonia levels (lactulose) in encephalopathy usually from lever failure
- Memorable Side Effects: Elevated magnesium (MOM), loose stools
- Watch out for accumulation in CKD (magnesium) – usually not an issue if used infrequently
- Can be used as needed
- Higher doses (lactulose) normally used for treatment of elevated ammonia
- Electrolyte imbalances (promotes fluid loss) possible but pretty unlikely unless prolonged, frequent use

Leukotriene Receptor Blocker

Example: Montelukast (Singulair)

Mechanism of Action: Blocks leukotriene receptors which can help reduce inflammation

NAPLEX Nuggets:
- Common Uses: asthma, allergic rhinitis
- Memorable Side Effects: Pretty well tolerated; Rare – psychiatric or unusual behavior changes
- Usually dosed in the evening, however in patients with ONLY allergies, they may give it at the time of day that works the best
- This medication is meant to control asthma, NOT provide acute relief with an exacerbation (albuterol is used for an asthma attack)
- Rare post-marketing case reports of neuropsychiatric problems (abnormal behavior, aggression, depression etc.)

Lipid Agents – Fibric Acid

Example: Gemfibrozil (Lopid), Fenofibrate (Tricor, Lofibra)

Mechanism of Action: Not well understood, ultimately decreases cholesterol, particularly used for triglycerides

NAPLEX Nuggets:
- Common Uses: Elevated Lipids (triglycerides)
- Memorable Side Effects: Dyspepsia (GI), rhabdomyolysis/myopathy possible especially when co-administered with statins
- Interacts with many of the statins, but sometimes used together (gemfibrozil)
- Important to educate patients, have heightened monitoring for statin adverse effects if using gemfibrozil with a statin

Loop Diuretics

Example: Furosemide (Lasix), Torsemide (Demedex), Bumetinide (Bumex), Ethacrynic Acid

Mechanism of Action: Inhibit sodium and chloride reabsorption in the ascending "Loop" of Henle in the kidney

NAPLEX Nuggets:

- Common Use: edema, hypertension, heart failure
- Memorable Side Effects: frequent urination, electrolyte depletion, low blood pressure, dehydration and renal impairment
- While loops can cause significant reductions in magnesium, calcium, sodium etc., potassium is one of the most important electrolytes to monitor and often patients require potassium supplementation; this can sometimes be offset by potassium sparing diuretics like spironolactone, ARBs like losartan, and ACE inhibitors like Lisinopril (all potentially increase potassium)
- Normal range for potassium: 3.5-5.1 (depending upon the lab)
- Frequent urination is a problem, make sure they are not being given too close to bedtime (if possible)
- Classic causes of edema include calcium channel blockers, pioglitazone, pregabalin, and NSAIDs.
- Loops deplete volume in the body, so patients run the risk of not having adequate perfusion through the kidney; elevations in creatinine from baseline can help us monitor for this risk
- Kidney function and electrolytes are going to be the primary labs to monitor
- Urinary output and monitoring of weights can be very important patient factors to monitor and help assess the efficacy of how well the loop diuretic (or any diuretic) is working

- If allergic to "sulfa" group, ethacrynic acid is still an option

Macrolide Antibiotics

Example: Erythromycin (Ery-tab), Azithromycin (Zithromax), Clarithromycin (Biaxin), Telithromycin (Ketek)

Mechanism of Action: Inhibits protein synthesis in bacteria

NAPLEX Nuggets:

- Common Uses: Upper respiratory i.e. ear infection, pneumonia, bronchitis, sinusitis; also used at lower doses chronically for gastroparesis (erythromycin)
- Memorable Side Effects: GI most common; QTc prolongation possible (very rare)
- Azithromycin is a common alternative to amoxicillin in pediatrics (ear infection, bronchitis, etc.)
- Numerous drug interactions via CYP3A4 (azithromycin has less), erythromycin, clarithromycin rarely used as an antibiotic due to this reason
- Clarithromycin may be part of H. Pylori (common cause of GI ulcer) regimen
- Dosed multiple times per day (except azithromycin much simpler dosing)
- If see erythromycin used chronically at low doses, likely being used to improve gastroparesis (slow GI motility common with diabetes)
- Telithromycin virtually never used due to hepatotoxicity risk

Monoamine Oxidase Inhibitors (MAOI's)

Example: Phenelzine (Nardil), Rasagiline (Azilect), Selegiline (Eldepryl)

Mechanism of Action: Blocks the enzyme monoamine oxidase which breaks down norepinephrine, dopamine and serotonin

NAPLEX Nuggets:
- Notorious for food interactions containing tyramine (cheese, beer, wine etc.)
- Use is very limited due to the drug/food interaction (especially for depression as there are so many other alternatives)
- Selegiline and Rasagiline are more selective for MAO Type B – used to prevent the breakdown of dopamine in Parkinson's
- Selegiline does come in a patch for depression (Emsam) – very expensive
- Risk of serotonin syndrome when used with SSRI's, TCA's etc.

Mood Stabilizer, Antimanic Agent

Example: Lithium (Lithobid)

Mechanism of Action: Not well understood

NAPLEX Nuggets:
- Common Uses: Acute and maintenance treatment for bipolar disorder
- Memorable Side Effects: Ataxia, CNS, depression, GI, tremor, hypothyroid, decreased creatinine clearance
- Early toxicity signs – nausea, vomiting, sedation, weakness, difficulty walking or coordinating movements, tremor
- Risk of seizure/coma with very high levels
- Kidney function very important to monitor
- Can impact Thyroid function (monitor TSH)
- Usually therapeutic level considered 0.5-1.2 mEq/L
- Classic drug interaction with thiazides, NSAIDs

Muscle Relaxants

Example: Carisoprodol (Soma), Cyclobenzaprine (Flexeril), Baclofen (Lioresal), Methocarbamol (Robaxin)

Mechanism of Action: Acts in the CNS and produces muscle relaxation

NAPLEX Nuggets:

- Common Uses: Muscle spasms, pain
- Memorable Side Effects: Anticholinergic activity, sedation, fall risk, confusion
- Normally used to relax the muscles in the case of muscle spasms, ideally this medication only needs to be used for a short period of time
- Elderly may particularly be at risk for side effects like anticholinergic effects, sedation, dizziness (fall risk)
- Onset of action is pretty quick (around an hour) so can be used on an as needed basis
- With the sedation side effect, we always need to caution our patients about driving, using machinery, etc.
- Dry mouth is common especially with frequent use
- On the Beer's list (avoid in the elderly if possible)

Nasal Corticosteroids

Example: Fluticasone (Flonase), Beclomethasone (Beconase AQ), Budesonide (Rhinocort), Mometasone (Nasonex)

Mechanism of Action: Nasal steroid that helps to reduce inflammation

NAPLEX Nuggets:
- Common Uses: Allergies
- Memorable Side Effects: Pretty well tolerated, likely nasal irritation, possible nose bleeds if any
- Gently shake the product for nasal inhalation and you may need to prime the nasal delivery device if it is the first time using it
- Educate patients that it may not work right away, it may take a few hours or up to a day or two to start working (because of this, it may not be the ideal to use this as needed, but I've certainly seen it prescribed this way before)
- It may only be necessary to use this medication seasonally based upon timing and duration of allergy symptoms
- Be sure to educate patients to clean the tip of the nasal delivery device as it can get pretty nasty!

Nicotine Replacement

Example: Nicotine gum, patches, lozenges, inhaler, nasal spray (Nicorette, Nicoderm, Commit, etc.)

Mechanism of Action: Replaces nicotine that would normally be ingested via smoking or chewing tobacco

NAPLEX Nuggets:
- Generally the first line therapy for smoking cessation
- Gums, inhalers, lozenges, nasal spray are intended for the as needed urge for smoking
- Patches are used more for daily control with more long acting effects
- When ingested (non patch formulation) they can cause some mouth/throat/GI irritation
- Recommended to completely stop smoking when using these products
- Patches can be worn for 24 hours
- Patches not meant to be cut, and only recommended to wear one at a time
- Considered a hazardous agent by the Environmental Protection Agency

Non Steroidal Anti-Inflammatory Drugs (NSAIDs)

Example(s): Ibuprofen (Advil, Motrin), Naproxen (Naprosyn, Aleve), Aspirin (Ecotrin), Diclofenac (Voltaren), Etodolac (Lodine), Indomethacin (Indocin), Ketorolac (Toradol), Meloxicam (Mobic), Nabumetone (Relafen), Oxaprozin (Daypro), Piroxicam (Feldene), Sulindac (Clinoril)

Mechanism of Action:

NAPLEX Nuggets:
- GI Bleeding and stomach upset (if drug necessary long term may need to add H2 blocker or PPI) – be very cautious in patients already receiving anticoagulation and/or antiplatelet medications
- Take with food
- Can exacerbate CHF (keep an eye out for increasing diuretic needs if NSAID started or increased)
- Kidney function needs to be monitored (diuretics, ACE inhibitors can increase risk of ARF)
- NSAIDs can exacerbate hypertension
- Drug(s) of choice for acute relief inflammation/pain in RA versus acetaminophen
- Usually second line for osteoarthritis (acetaminophen first line)
- Not the safest pain/fever reliever in the elderly (typically acetaminophen is safer)
- Not used in pregnancy for pain/headache
- Ibuprofen commonly used in pediatrics (4-10 mg/kg/dose)
- Ibuprofen and naproxen are available over the counter
- Indomethacin is used for gout flares
- Ketorolac has a boxed warning for GI bleed (recommends use no longer than 5 days

- Of the really common NSAIDs, ibuprofen has a shorter half life than naproxen and meloxicam so it needs to be dosed more frequently
- Due to effects on platelets, NSAIDs are typically held before/after surgery to reduce the risk of bleeding; also monitor for bruising
- Avoid Aspirin in pediatrics – risk of Reye's syndrome
- Baby Aspirin (sometimes 325 mg) used for stroke/MI prevention
- Toxicity can cause tinnitus - ringing in the ears (Aspirin in particular)

Norepinephrine Reuptake Inhibitor

Example: Atomoxetine (Strattera)

Mechanism of Action: Inhibits reuptake of norepinephrine

NAPLEX Nuggets:
- Common Uses: ADHD
- Memorable Side Effects: sweating, dry mouth, GI, increase BP, weight loss
- Non-controlled substance used for ADHD is the big advantage of atomoxetine compared to methylphenidate, amphetamine salts, etc.
- Special warning regarding increased risk of suicidal thoughts and behaviors
- Can increase BP, cardiovascular problems, and increase risk of poor appetite/weight loss just like tradition stimulants (methylphenidate)

NRTI (Nucleoside Reverse Transcriptase Inhibitor), Antiretroviral

Example: Abacavir (Ziagen), Didanosine (Videx), Emtricitabine (Emtriva), Lamivudine (Epivir), Zidovudine (Retrovir)

Mechanism of Action: Blocks DNA polymerase action and stops viral replication

NAPLEX Nuggets:
- Incredibly important that patients remain adherent to HIV therapy as a resistance is a major problem
- Fat redistribution (lipodystrophy) is a possible adverse effect, example – "buffalo hump"
- Boxed warning for lactic acidosis and fatty liver
- HIV drugs from different classes are utilized together to maximize therapy and minimize resistance
- GI side effects are most common

NRTI (Nucleotide Reverse Transcriptase Inhibitor), Antiretroviral

Example: Tenofovir (Viread)

Mechanism of Action: Stops the action of HBV polymerase in the treatment of Hep B, and interferes with DNA Polymerase in treatment of HIV

NAPLEX Nuggets:
- Adherence very important in HIV therapy
- Similar adverse effect profile in many ways to the nucleoside analogs
- Boxed warning for lactic acidosis/fatty liver
- GI adverse effects
- Increase in cholesterol possible
- May decrease bone mineral density

Ophthalmic antihistamine

Example: Olopatadine (Patanol)

Mechanism of Action: Histamine receptor blocker (eye drops)

NAPLEX Nuggets:
- Common Uses: Allergies where eyes are affected
- Memorable Side Effects: eye irritation
- Blocks histamine receptors, so dry eye is a possibility
- At least 5 minutes between other eye drops is ideal
- May only need to use this medication seasonally depending upon allergies

Opioids

Example: Hydromorphone (Dilaudid), Codeine, Oxycodone (Oxycontin), Morphine (MS Contin), Oxycodone (Oxycontin), Fentanyl (Duragesic), Hydrocodone with Acetaminophen (Vicodin, Norco), Methadone (Dolophine), Tramadol (Ultram)

Mechanism of Action: Binds opioid receptors inhibiting CNS pain pathways and causes pain relief

NAPLEX Nuggets:
- Common Uses: Management of pain disorders, both chronic and acute
- Memorable Side Effects: Constipation, sedation, CNS effects like confusion, delirium etc., respiratory depression
- Most are a scheduled 2 controlled substance; risk of addiction, dependence, etc. (exception Tylenol with Codeine – schedule 3, Tramadol – schedule 4)
- It is critical to educate/assess patients for constipation if they are taking frequent opioids
- Naloxone (Narcan) is reversal agent for opioids
- Driving/working machinery is certainly risky when using opioids as they can cause significant sedation (usually patients get used to this side effect if they take the medication chronically)
- Tramadol can increase seizure risk
- Often used in combo with acetaminophen, be sure to educate about acetaminophen toxicity as dosing increases and use of other agents that contain acetaminophen – oxycodone, codeine, hydrocodone
- MS Contin and Oxycontin are the brand names for long acting morphine and oxycodone respectively
- Remember that long acting opioids should NOT be used as needed (Oxycontin, MS Contin, Fentanyl patches)

- Morphine has the most available dosage forms – suppository, injectable, oral tablet, long acting, liquid etc.
- At higher doses, risk of withdrawal is high if abruptly discontinued
- No maximum dose except for if it contains acetaminophen! Tramadol does have a max, risk of seizures especially above therapeutic doses
- Methadone is a pain to convert to/from
- Methadone maintenance program for addicts requires special licensing, using methadone for pain management does not
- Opioid Conversion Information http://www.globalrph.com/narcotic.htm
- In most cases, flushing fentanyl patches is appropriate (risk of pets, children getting them out of garbage and overdosing)

Oxazolidinones (Antibiotic)

Example: Linezolid (Zyvox)

Mechanism of Action: Binds to the 50S subunit via 23S ribosomal RNA and inhibits the 70S formation which is necessary for replication

NAPLEX Nuggets:
- Activity against resistant/troublesome bugs like MRSA (methicillin resistant staph aureus) and VRE (Vancomycin resistant enterococcus)
- MAOI activity so may need to hold or adjust antidepressants that can increase serotonin (SSRI's, TCA's etc.)
- Oral and IV available
- Expensive
- Rare AE's like myelosuppression (bone marrow suppression, low WBC etc.) and lactic acidosis

PDE-5 inhibitor

Example: Sildenafil (Viagra), Tadalafil (Cialis), Vardenafil (Levitra)

Mechanism of Action: Phosphodiesterase Type 5 inhibitor – releases nitric oxide which is necessary for erection

NAPLEX Nuggets:
- Common Uses: Erectile dysfunction, pulmonary arterial hypertension
- Memorable Side Effects: Low blood pressure, vision color changes (seeing blue tinges in vision), flushing
- Originally developed as a blood pressure medication; caution patients about risk of low blood pressure
- Drug interaction with systemic nitrate/nitroglycerine products (advise patients about potential interaction and elevated risk of low blood pressure)
- Be sure to assess if other medications may be contributing to sexual dysfunction (antidepressants like SSRI's are a classic example)
- Medications in this class can be given daily or as needed

Penicillin Type Antibiotics

Example: Amoxicillin (Amoxil), Amoxicillin/Clavulanate (Augmentin), Penicillin, Ampicillin or Ampicillin/Sulbactam (Unasyn), Piperacillin/Tazobactam (Zosyn)

Mechanism of Action: Inhibits bacterial cell wall formation

NAPLEX Nuggets:

- Common Uses: (Amoxicillin or Amox/Clav) Ear infection, sinusitis, strep throat, skin infections
- Amoxicillin usually first line in pediatrics for ear infection at 80-90 mg/kg
- Pip/Tazo (IV only) has really broad coverage especially beneficial for pseudomonas (nasty, resistant hospital infection) - Pseudomonas has a characteristic "sweet" smell
- Memorable Side Effects: GI side effects most common, allergy, rash
- Many patients have an allergy to penicillin; these medications are all from the same class and should not be used in patients with a severe allergy (if it is an intolerance like stomach upset, it may be prudent to try a "penicillin" type antibiotic again depending upon the patient's situation and other antibiotics available for use)
- Diarrhea and GI upset are going to be the major/common side effects with this class; with mild GI upset and/or diarrhea, hopefully the patient can tough it out and continue therapy
- Giving amoxicillin with food or a snack may help reduce GI upset
- We are going to want to monitor the response of the patient, hopefully they will begin feeling better at least by day 2 or 3 of treatment
- Temperature would be an important thing to monitor for patients who were significantly febrile

- If suspension is used (common in pediatrics), you must adequately shake to disperse the medication!

Phosphate Binders

Example: Calcium Acetate (Phoslo), Sevelamer (Renagel, Renvela), Aluminum Hydroxide

Mechanism of Action: Binds with dietary phosphate in the gut and gets excreted in the feces leading to lower phosphate levels

NAPLEX Nuggets:
- Short term use only of aluminum based phosphate binders is recommended to avoid aluminum toxicity
- Memorable Side Effects: Hypercalcemia (calcium acetate), GI (N/V/D)
- Used as a phosphate binder usually in CKD as phosphate levels can build up in end stage renal disease
- Dosed with meals
- Need to watch calcium as this medication can increase levels (calcium acetate)
- Sevelamer an option in a patient with already high calcium levels (non-calcium based)

Platinum Drugs

Example: Carboplatin, Cisplatin

Mechanism of Action: Disrupts and changes the double helix, forms DNA cross links

NAPLEX Nuggets:
- Very high incidence of chemotherapy induced nausea and vomiting
- Neuropathy
- Monitor WBC, ANC etc., risk of suppression and infection
- Nephrotoxicity, kidney function monitoring important
- Ototoxicity
- If anaphylactic or hypersensitivity reaction, may see epinephrine, steroids, and/or diphenhydramine

Potassium Sparing Diuretic, Miscellaneous

Example: Triamterene often in combo with HCTZ (Dyazide)

Mechanism of Action: Triamterene is a potassium sparing diuretic that blocks sodium channels in the kidney

NAPLEX Nuggets:
- Common Uses: Hypertension, edema
- Memorable Side Effects: Triamterene (hyperkalemia), dehydration (rising creatinine and BUN), low blood pressure, orthostasis risk, electrolyte imbalances
- Much like all diuretics, in relation to the effects on the kidney, the risk of overdiuresis is worsening kidney function
- We can often reduce the potassium supplementation (especially patients on high doses of KCl supplements) burden by using potassium sparing diuretics
- Triamterene, while generally lumped into the group of potassium sparing diuretics because it causes elevations in potassium, does have a slightly different mechanism of action – it acts on sodium channels in the late distal convoluted tubule; it doesn't compete with aldosterone like spironolactone
- Patients often forget they are actually on two medications when they are used in combination in one pill
- See HCTZ (hydrochlorothiazide) alone for its clinical pearls

Potassium Supplement

Example: Potassium Chloride (Klor-Con, K-Dur)

Mechanism of Action: Replaces body's potassium

NAPLEX Nuggets:

- Common Uses: Low potassium, diuretic use
- Memorable Side Effects: GI side effects (oral), hyperkalemia
- High risk electrolyte as hyperkalemia can cause cardiac arrhythmias
- Often supplementation is necessary in patients who are on diuretics like furosemide (except potassium sparing diuretics which can increase potassium levels)
- GI upset is most common and best to take with food
- With the wax-matrix formulation of potassium, patients may find the outer coating remaining in their stool; the drug is designed to leak out of the matrix shell, educate them that they are getting their potassium (i.e. this is normal and not an issue)
- Normal potassium level: 3.5-5.1 mEq/L (may vary slightly depending upon lab)
- By adding ACE Inhibitors, ARBs, or potassium sparing diuretics to the patients medication regimen, we may be able to get away with less potassium supplement
- Sodium polystyrene sulfonate - Kayexalate (antidote) is used to treat hyperkalemia, insulin may also be utilized in emergency

Prostaglandin, Ophthalmic

Example: Bimatoprost (Lumigan), Latanoprost (Xalatan), Travoprost (Travatan)

Mechanism of Action: Prostaglandin F2 alpha analog – decreases intraocular pressure

NAPLEX Nuggets:
- Common Uses: Glaucoma
- Memorable Side Effects: Change in eye color, eye irritation
- Generally dosed in the evening for glaucoma
- Change in eye color may be permanent (change to brown)
- Many glaucoma patients will be on multiple eye drops – at least 5 minutes is the appropriate amount of time to wait between drops
- Latanoprost expires in 42 days once removed from the fridge (REFRIDGERATE until put into use!)

Protease Inhibitors

Example: Atazanavir (Reyataz), Darunavir (Prezista), Fosamprenavir (Lexiva), Indinavir (Crixivan), Lopinavir/Ritonavir (Kaletra), Saquinavir (Invirase), Tipranavir (Aptivus)

Mechanism of Action: Inhibits viral protease activity which results in deformed viral particles, used to treat HIV

NAPLEX Nuggets:
- Can cause abnormal fat distribution (lipodystrophy), increased cholesterol, triglycerides – "Buffalo hump"
- Hyperglycemia
- Tons of drug interactions (primarily via CYP3A4)
- Rash
- Ritonavir used to inhibit CYP3A4 which increases concentrations of Lopinavir when used in combination
- Adherence/compliance critical with all HIV medications as HIV mutates quickly

Proton Pump Inhibitor

Example: Omeprazole (Prilosec), Pantoprazole (Protonix), Lansoprazole (Prevacid), Esomeprazole (Nexium), Rabeprazole (Aciphex), Dexlansoprazole (Dexilant)

Mechanism of Action: Inhibits proton pumps in the stomach leading to a less acidic environment

NAPLEX Nuggets:

- Common Uses: GERD, ulcer, Barrett's esophagus
- Memorable Side Effects: Usually pretty well tolerated; Long term use: Possibility to increase fracture risk, decrease B12 levels, C. diff risk, low magnesium
- PPI's are the most potent acid blocker on the market
- PPI's are generally dosed 30 minutes or so before meals – this is a recommendation, not an absolute (example if a patient likes to get up and eat right away upon rising, the medication will still likely be beneficial, but may not have a maximal effect)
- For some patients PPI's may not work very quickly, i.e. it might take a few days for maximal effect
- For the above reason, as needed (PRN) PPI's can possibly be effective, but are generally not used
- Use short term if possible due to increased risk of osteoporosis, C. Diff, low magnesium, and B12 deficiency if used long term
- Barrett's esophagus, high risk GI medications (i.e. NSAIDs, prednisone), or chronic GI bleed are examples where patients may require indefinite therapy
- If GI bleed is problematic, monitoring hemoglobin and/or hemoccult (blood in the stool) might be appropriate to assess possible blood loss

Quinolone Antibiotics

Example: Levofloxacin (Levaquin), Ciprofloxacin (Cipro), Moxifloxacin (Avelox)

Mechanism of Action: Inhibits bacterial DNA synthesis

NAPLEX Nuggets:
- Common Uses: UTI's (Cipro, Levaquin), Pneumonia (Levaquin, Avelox)
- Memorable Side Effects: GI side effects, QTc prolongation (rare)
- Commonly used for the treatment of UTI's; great coverage against many gram negative bacteria
- Dose adjustments might be necessary in patients with poor kidney function (exception Avelox)
- Should not be co-administered with iron or calcium products as this can significant reduce absorption and possibly lead to treatment failure
- Ciprofloxacin generally NOT used for pneumonia (Other quinolones like levofloxacin and moxifloxacin can be) – has poor activity against Strep. pneumoniae (a common cause of pneumonia)
- Cipro usually has to be dosed multiple times per day (at least twice)
- Spontaneous tendon rupture has been reported with quinolones (extremely rare)
- Can interact with warfarin and raise INR

Reverse Transcriptase Inhibitor – Non-nucleoside

Example: Efavirenz (Sustiva), Delavirdine (Rescriptor), Etravirine (Intelence), Rilprivirine (Edurant)

Mechanism of Action: Inhibits reverse transcriptase, but is considered a non-nucleoside medication

NAPLEX Nuggets:
- CNS side effects and psychiatric changes (abnormal dreams, hallucinations, etc.)
- Hepatotoxicity
- Rash – can continue if mild, but DC if severe
- Caution in seizure disorder

Selective Estrogen Receptor Modulator

Example: Raloxifene (Evista), Tamoxifen (Soltamox)

Mechanism of Action: Has blocking activity at some estrogen receptors and agonist activity at other estrogen receptors

NAPLEX Nuggets:

- Raloxifene is indicated for osteoporosis as well as breast cancer (prevention only)
- Tamoxifen is indicated for the treatment of breast cancer
- Tamoxifen length of use is usually reassessed in 5 years and may be done prior to an aromatase inhibitor like anastrozole or letrozole
- Increases risk of DVT
- Adverse effects of hot flashes, change in menses (pre-menopausal), mood changes etc.

Selective Serotonin Reuptake Inhibitors

Example: Citalopram (Celexa), Sertraline (Zoloft), Paroxetine (Paxil), Fluoxetine (Prozac), Fluvoxamine (Luvox), Escitalopram (Lexapro)

Mechanism of Action: Selective serotonin reuptake inhibitor; increases serotonin in the brain

NAPLEX Nuggets:
- Common Uses: Depression, anxiety, PTSD
- Memorable Side Effects: GI side effects (N/V/D), can really cause sedation or activation depending upon the patient, changes in mental status, hyponatremia (rare)
- The dose of citalopram should be limited/monitored closely in the elderly as well as patients on omeprazole (recommended max citalopram of 20 mg/day)
- SSRI's are generally considered the first line medication to treat depression, they are usually well tolerated, and less risky than the TCA's in the situation of suicide by overdosing on pills
- Stomach/GI complaints/diarrhea are probably the most common SE's
- There may be an increased risk of suicidal thinking when first starting these medications (there is a BOXED warning for this risk)
- Although not terribly common, hyponatremia (low sodium) is a possible unique side effect with SSRI's and much more likely in patients already prone to hyponatremia – classic example would be patients who are taking diuretics, which can also lower sodium
- Remember that these drugs are not an immediate fix! In most cases, SSRI's take weeks sometimes months before a patient will start improving; however side effects will be apparent from the start of the medication, making it difficult to coach our patients to

continue the medication in the first few weeks after starting it

- SSRI's are used in pregnancy, but the risk versus the benefit needs to be assessed on a case by case basis
- SSRI's can decrease libido

Serotonin and Norepinephrine Reuptake Inhibitors (SNRI)

Example: Duloxetine (Cymbalta), Venlafaxine (Effexor), Desvenlafaxine (Pristiq)

Mechanism of Action: Serotonin and norepinephrine reuptake inhibitor (SNRI)

NAPLEX Nuggets:
- Common Uses: Depression, pain syndromes, fibromyalgia
- Memorable Side Effects: GI side effects, can exacerbate hypertension (usually at higher doses), CNS changes
- Has effects on both serotonin and norepinephrine
- Indicated to help with pain syndromes as well depression; neuropathic pain in particular is where you will likely see it used most frequently
- GI and central nervous system side effects (CNS) will likely be the most common
- Decreased libido can be an issue for patients taking and SNRI
- Be careful with the risk of serotonin syndrome especially in patients on other serotonergic medications

Short Acting Beta Agonists

Example: Albuterol (Proventil HFA, ProAir HFA, Ventolin HFA), Levalbuterol (Xopenex)

Mechanism of Action: Stimulates beta-2 receptors leading to relaxation of smooth muscle and opening of airways

NAPLEX Nuggets:

- This class is the mainstay for an acute asthma exacerbation...i.e. it has a rapid onset and can begin to open up the airway in a few short minutes
- It is often used with ipratropium (Duoneb/Combivent = brand name)
- Remember that albuterol (a beta agonist) will have opposite effects of Beta-blockers! Instead of reduced pulse, you could see tachycardia
- Too much beta-agonist can also be a potential cause of tremor/shakiness
- In patients who are taking multiple inhaled respiratory medications at the same time, albuterol will be done first to help open up the airways
- With patients who are frequently using their albuterol inhaler (or nebs) or presenting to the emergency room, make sure that they are reassessed to have their controller (usually inhaled corticosteroids, long acting beta agonists, Montelukast etc.) medication adjusted
- General guide for "uncontrolled asthma", remember the rule of "2" – Use of rescue inhaler (albuterol) more than 2x/week, nighttime symptoms more than 2x/month, greater than 2 canisters of albuterol/year
- Albuterol found in combo with ipratropium (Respimat, Duoneb)
- Very important to assess technique of administration if patients present with frequent refills or states ineffectiveness of medication

Smoking Cessation Agent, Nicotine Partial Agonist

Example: Varenicline (Chantix)

Mechanism of Action: Partial agonist at nicotine receptors (blocks craving/positive response from nicotine)

NAPLEX Nuggets:

- Common Uses: Smoking cessation
- Memorable Side Effects: Abnormal dreams, insomnia, GI, mental health concerns
- Abnormal behavioral and psych issues is a significant problem
- Vivid or unusual dreams is a concern for patients
- Box warning for depression/suicide, etc.
- Recommended only to use for 11 weeks
- Intended to make smoking less rewarding/enjoyable
- Generally start this medication a week before scheduled quit date

Sodium-Glucose Cotransporter 2 Inhibitors (SGLT2)

Example: Canagliflozin (Invokana), Dapagliflozin (Farxiga), Empagliflozin (Jardiance)

Mechanism of Action: Blocks SGLT-2 which results in elimination of glucose in the urine and reduction of blood glucose

NAPLEX Nuggets:

- Warning on Ketoacidosis with use of SGLT-2 inhibitors
- Need to monitor potassium as these drugs can increase potassium (pay attention to patients already on ACE, K+ sparing diuretics etc.)
- Risk of urinary tract infections/candida – remember that more sugar (glucose) in the urine = more food for bugs to utilize
- Kidney function monitoring important
- Low blood sugar risk particularly with other drugs like sulfonylureas
- Bone fracture risk
- Be on the lookout for low BP/volume depletion – elderly, patient on diuretics may be at greater risk

Statins

Example: Atorvastatin (Lipitor), Simvastatin (Zocor), Rosuvastatin (Crestor), Lovastatin (Mevacor), Fluvastatin (Lescol), Pravastatin (Pravachol), Pitavastatin (Livalo)

Mechanism of Action: HMG Co-A reductase inhibitor (causes decrease in LDL)

NAPLEX Nuggets:
- Common Uses: Reduction of cholesterol (particularly LDL)
- Memorable Side Effects: muscle aches, rhabdomyolysis (rare but serious)
- Statins like atorvastatin are one of the mainstays of therapy to reduce cholesterol, and more particularly LDL (bad cholesterol)
- The most notable side effect with statins that you will likely hear patients complain about is myopathy (muscle aches/pain)
- Usually muscle aches are all over which can help you differentiate from other pain conditions or pain/soreness from an injury or overuse
- Liver toxicity is very rare, FDA put out a release saying that routine monitoring is not necessary anymore
- Contraindicated in pregnancy
- Patients who do not tolerate one statin, may try another statin as long as adverse effects aren't too severe (i.e. rhabdomyolysis); if you notice that the patient had an allergy or intolerance, you need to clarify with the patient/provider
- CPK will be the primary lab to test for rhabdomyolysis – breakdown of muscle; this elevation in CPK may eventually lead to kidney failure
- If they are going to, patients usually will present with myopathy when the medication is first started or increased, but be on the lookout for new medications

that can interact with statins like CYP3A4 inhibitor drug interactions with medications like fluconazole or erythromycin (this will cause many statin concentrations in the body to go up potentially leading to toxicity)

- Gemfibrozil is a cholesterol medication that also interacts with atorvastatin – this drug interaction should be addressed with the primary provider
- Simvastatin dose of 80 mg is no longer recommended
- Important dose restrictions on simvastatin due to drug interactions with amlodipine, amiodarone, verapamil, diltiazem
- For many of the older statins it is "recommended" to give them at night – the theory is cholesterol production happens at night (newer statins it is not specified – i.e. pitavastatin, rosuvastatin, atorvastatin)
- Statin Intensity Chart:

Pharmacotherapy Options		
High Intensity Statin	Moderate Intensity Statin	Low Intensity Statin
Lowers LDL by ≥ 50%	Lowers LDL by 30 – 49%	Lowers LDL by < 30%
Atorvastatin (40) 80 mg Rosuvastatin 20-40 mg	Atorvastatin 10-20 mg Rosuvastatin 5-10 mg Simvastatin 20-40 mg Pravastatin 40-80 mg Lovastatin 40 mg Fluvastatin 40 mg twice daily Fluvastatin XL 80 mg Pitavastatin 2-4 mg	Simvastatin 10 mg Pravastatin 10-20 mg Lovastatin 20 mg Fluvastatin 20-40 mg Pitavastatin 1 mg

- Multiple factors go into selecting whether a patient is a candidate for statin therapy; diabetes, smoking, age,

gender, race, hypertension – Here's a risk calculator
http://tools.acc.org/ASCVD-Risk-Estimator/

Stimulant Laxatives

Example: Bisacodyl (Dulcolax), Sennosides (Senna)

Mechanism of Action: Stimulates GI movement by irritating smooth muscle

NAPLEX Nuggets:
- Common Uses: Constipation
- Memorable Side Effects: Abdominal pain
- Used to promote bowel movement
- Similar medication class as Sennosides, but Bisacodyl has a suppository formulation
- Suppository formulation is nice for patients who may have difficulty swallowing/can't take oral
- Can be used as needed
- Often used in treatment/prevention of opioid induced constipation
- Senna-S product contains docusate (a stool softener as well as the stimulant)

Systemic Corticosteroids

Example: Budesonide (Entocort), Prednisone (Deltasone), Dexamethasone, Methylprednisolone (Medrol), Prednisolone (Orapred)

Mechanism of Action: Suppresses leukocytes and ultimately reduces inflammation, suppresses adrenal function and the immune system

NAPLEX Nuggets:

- Common Uses: Acute inflammatory states (dermatitis, arthritis flare, Crohn's, pneumonia, asthma exacerbation, etc.), immunosuppressant
- Memorable Side Effects: GI side effects, insomnia, hyperglycemia, long term use; suppress immune system, increase osteoporosis risk as well as cause adrenal insufficiency
- Budesonide is usually specifically reserved for ulcerative colitis or Crohn's disease
- Be sure to take steroids with food as they can be pretty hard on the GI tract
- In patients with diabetes, educate them that a fluctuation in blood sugars may occur when starting, changing doses, or discontinuing this medication due to the adverse effect of hyperglycemia
- Long term corticosteroid use can lead to increased risk Cushing's (moon face), diabetes, and osteoporosis; make sure long term use is assessed frequently to minimize length and dose of steroids
- In patients on long term use, they should be assessed if vitamin D and/or calcium and bisphosphonates should be added to reduce osteoporosis risk
- Insomnia is common in the short term, but may resolve as short term use goes to longer term use

- Short "bursts" 3 days to a week or 2 are often used to relieve acute inflammatory states causing patient distress (asthma, rheumatoid arthritis, etc.)
- Corticosteroids (especially long term and higher doses) can also suppress the immune system
- Alternative to NSAIDs in acute gout or rheumatoid arthritis flare

Taxanes

Example: Docetaxel (Taxotere), Paclitaxel

Mechanism of Action: Multiple mechanisms, but primarily stabilizes the microtubules stopping the cell cycle

NAPLEX Nuggets:
- Hypersensitivity reaction possible and pretreatment with steroids may be necessary
- Very high incidence of neuropathy
- Fluid retention possible
- Stomatitis
- Hair loss
- WBC, ANC etc. is very important to monitor as these drugs suppress the immune system

Tetracycline Antibiotics

Example: Doxycycline (Vibramycin), Tetracycline, Minocycline (Minocin), Demclocycine

Mechanism of Action: Inhibits bacterial protein synthesis

NAPLEX Nuggets:

- Common Uses: Often an alternative to penicillin antibiotics (skin infections, pneumonia, etc.), SIADH (Hyponatremia) - demeclocycline
- Memorable Side Effects: GI side effects, photosensitivity, rash
- May give with meals if GI upset is a problem
- Can cause birth defects (category D)
- Can make patients more susceptible to sunburn
- Possibility to cause tooth discoloration (usually long term use only or multiple courses)
- Avoid timing calcium, iron, antacids at the same time (may block absorption and decrease amount of drug absorbed)

Thiazide Like Diuretics

Example: Indapamide, Metolazone (Zaroxolyn)

Mechanism of Action: Increases excretion of sodium, water, potassium via blockade of sodium reabsorption in the distal tubules

NAPLEX Nuggets:

- Works similar to thiazide diuretics, but has a different structure (the reason why they are called "thiazide like" or "thiazide related")
- Potassium depletion is possible, especially in patients who may be on loops as well (most often used in CHF to promote fluid loss)
- Similar effects to loops with the exception that thiazide like diuretics may increase calcium versus deplete calcium
- Monitor kidney function – dehydration (rising BUN and Creatinine will be important to follow) possible with the loss of fluid
- Metolazone likely more effective when baseline kidney function is already poor (compared with hydrochlorothiazide)
- Can increase uric acid
- Frequent urination

Thrombolytics

Example: Alteplase (Activase, tPA)

Mechanism of Action: Binds to fibrin and breaks up blood clots

NAPLEX Nuggets:

- Common Uses: Stroke, Pulmonary embolism, MI when PCI not appropriate or not possible, also can be used to open up central venous access (Cathflo)
- The sooner the better in an acute ischemic event!
- Need to use this medication quickly at onset of stroke to have maximal benefit
- Classified as a thrombolytic (clot buster)
- Bleed risk is important to monitor – low chance of causing intracranial bleeding, but not good if this happens
- Extra caution if patients are already receiving anticoagulants (warfarin, dabigatran, etc.)
- Need to monitor for high blood pressure or other condition that might increase the risk of bleeding

Thyroid Replacement

Example: Levothyroxine (Synthroid, Levothroid)

Mechanism of Action: Synthetic T4 hormone, converted to active T3 metabolite

NAPLEX Nuggets:

- Common Uses: Replacement hormone for patients with hypothyroidism
- Memorable Side Effects: anxiety, tachycardia, weight loss, decreased bone mineral density, insomnia, GI side effects
- Remember that in patients with hypothyroidism, they will have a lack of energy, fatigue, possible weight gain and many symptoms that might mimic depression
- If hypothyroidism causes fatigue and lethargy symptoms, remember that giving too much levothyroxine will cause the opposite (i.e. it will ramp up the patient putting them at risk for insomnia, tachycardia, anxiety etc.)
- TSH is the major monitoring parameter for levothyroxine dosing – Dosing is counterintuitive! Remember that when TSH is low, it indicates that levothyroxine should be decreased; the reason for this is due to a negative feedback loop
- In practice, I commonly see ½ tabs, and possibly alternating daily doses which can increase risk for errors and confusion
- Use of calcium, iron, and other cation supplements is extremely common – givin levothyroxine together will these can significantly block the absorption of the levothyroxine, and our patient may require an increase in their levothyroxine dose
- With administration of levothyroxine, it is generally recommended to give early in the morning prior to other meds/food etc. HOWEVER if a patient is stabilized

(TSH is normal) and doesn't take it this way, it is ok – consistency is the key!

- Usual TSH Range – 0.5-5
- Notorious medication causes of hypothyroidism: amiodarone and lithium

Topical Analgesic, Antiarrhythmic

Example: Lidocaine (Lidoderm, Xylocaine)

Mechanism of Action: Reduces conduction in the heart by preventing nerve impulses via reduction of membrane permeability to sodium ions, works similarly with analgesic effects topically – prevents nerve impulses

NAPLEX Nuggets:
- Analgesic effects are LOCAL, not systemic – so you apply lidocaine at the site of pain
- Often given with painful Rocephin injections to reduce pain
- 12 hours on/12 hours off is recommended with the patch formulation and can use up to 3 patches at a time
- As an antiarrhythmic, used in VFib or Vtach with no pulse (systemic)

Did you find this study guide beneficial? Please do me a HUGE favor and leave a kind review on Amazon! – Thanks in advance!

Topical Corticosteroids

Example: Clobetasol (Temovate), Hydrocortisone, Betamethasone (Diprolene), Fluocinolone (Synalar), Triamcinolone (Kenalog),

Mechanism of Action: Suppresses mediators of inflammation (histamine, kinins, prostaglandins etc.) resulting in less inflammation/redness

NAPLEX Nuggets:
- Common Uses: Dermatitis, psoriasis
- Memorable Side Effects: local irritation - systemic side effects can happen but rare; prolonged use, large areas increase systemic absorption and risk of adrenal suppression, HPA-axis suppression, etc.
- If patients don't see improvement in condition in 1-2 weeks, be sure they know to get reassessed
- Long term use, large quantities probably more concerning in young children
- Systemic problems not likely if used short term

Tri-Cyclic Antidepressants (TCA's)

Example: Amitriptyline (Elavil), Nortriptyline (Pamelor), Doxepin (Sinequan)

Mechanism of Action: Tri-cyclic antidepressant (highly anticholinergic) – inhibits reuptake of serotonin and possibly norepinephrine

NAPLEX Nuggets:
- Common Uses: Depression, neuropathy, pain syndromes, anxiety, PTSD, sleep, itch
- Memorable Side Effects: Anticholinergic + confusion, fall risk in elderly
- Anticholinergic effect = anti – SLUDs; can't salivate, lacrimate, urinate, or defecate OR can't spit, see, pee, or poop
- TCA's generally not recommended in the elderly due to anticholinergic effects
- In addition, cognitive impairment is not a good thing in the elderly due to possibility of preexisting dementia
- TCA's may have some benefit in neuropathy, generally cheaper than SNRI's (duloxetine) which can be also beneficial in neuropathy
- Not a good first line choice for sleep or depression (other agents exist that are much safer)
- Look out for TCA's causing the prescribing cascade! Artificial tears for dry eyes, constipation medications, BPH medications like tamsulosin, dementia medications, or artificial saliva
- Nortriptyline generally considered safer than amitriptyline in the elderly
- Doxepin often used to help with itching and/or sleep

Urinary Analgesic

Example: Phenazopyridine (Pyridium)

Mechanism of Action: Local anesthetic action in the bladder/urinary tract

NAPLEX Nuggets:
- Common Uses: Painful urination (dysuria)
- Memorable Side Effects: GI, dizziness (minimal)
- Very important to identify patients who are taking this and have them assessed for infection or something else going on
- Often will see it used short term for painful urination associated with UTI
- Not intended for long term use
- Ensure adequate fluid intake if patient is having UTI's and/or using this medication frequently
- Can accumulate in kidney disease

Vasoconstrictor

Example: Vasopressin (Vasostrict)

Mechanism of Action: Causes an increase in cyclic AMP which causes multiple effects including vasoconstriction

NAPLEX Nuggets:
- Common Uses: Vasodilation related shock
- Memorable Side Effects: Arrhythmia, MI, heart failure
- Vasoconstrictor used to increase BP (used for vasodilatory shock)
- Can impact sodium levels
- BP/Pulse important to monitor

Vasodilator, Antihypertensive (Non-Nitrate)

Example: Hydralazine (Apresoline)

Mechanism of Action: Directly dilates arteries and arterioles (decreases BP)

NAPLEX Nuggets:
- Common Uses: Hypertension
- Memorable Side Effects: Low BP, CNS changes, exacerbate/contribute to Lupus (rare)
- Fall/orthostatic blood pressure risk
- Dosed multiple times per day so difficult for patients to adhere to medication regimen

Vinca Alkaloids

Example: Vincristine (Vincasar), Vinblastine

Mechanism of Action: Tubulin binder which stops the cell cycle and further proliferation

NAPLEX Nuggets:
- Vesicant
- Be on the looking out for other drugs that can cause SIADH (carbamazepine, SSRI's etc.) as these medications can worsen SIADH
- Neuropathy is a common adverse effect
- Hair loss
- Be on the lookout for patients with gout as they can increase uric acid
- Obviously suppresses immune system, monitor WBC etc.

Vitamin D Derivative

Example: Vitamin D, ergocalciferol, cholecalciferol

Mechanism of Action: Vitamin D increases calcium/phosphorus absorption in the gut

NAPLEX Nuggets:

- Common Uses: Vitamin supplementation in osteoporosis or vitamin D deficiency (Rickets), hypoparathyroidism
- Memorable Side Effects: Well tolerated at replacement doses (can accumulate if high doses used for a long period of time – fat soluble)
- Most commonly used in patients with osteoporosis history
- Moving target on what is an adequate goal vitamin D level; 30 - 35 ng/mL range or greater
- Remember that patients in northern climates (less sunlight) may be at higher risk for low levels
- For maintenance, can simply do daily supplements at lower doses (i.e. 1,000 to 2,000 units), but may also do BIG doses once monthly (50,000 units)

Vitamin K Antagonist, Anticoagulant

Example: Warfarin (Coumadin, Jantoven)

Mechanism of Action: Inhibition of clotting factors 2, 7, 9, and 10 – some folks remember this by the term "SNOT" seven, nine, '10', two

NAPLEX Nuggets:

- Common Uses: Prevention of blood clots such as DVT, prevention of thromboembolic stroke from atrial fibrillation
- Common Side Effects: Bleeding, purple toe syndrome (rare)
- Warfarin has a ton of drug interactions, antibiotics (sulfamethoxazole/trimethoprim, metronidazole, levofloxacin etc.) being a very common cause of drug interactions; be sure physician is aware/reminded that patients are on warfarin when new medications are started or doses of medications might be changed
- Bleeding, Bruising, INR, CBC are of highest monitoring importance
- Vitamin K is the antidote to too much warfarin; ideal way to give vitamin K is orally – also remember that many foods contain vitamin K (green leafy vegetables etc.); diet changes can affect INR, consistency is the key!
- Younger patients may require doses 10+ mg or greater whereas elderly maybe need as little as 1-2 mg per day
- Usual goal range INR is 2-3; It is always important to have the goal INR range listed/addressed by the practitioner monitoring warfarin; this allows you to ask questions as to why the dose wasn't changed if the INR falls outside this range
- In patients who are at high risk for bleed, i.e. frequent falls, GI bleed history etc., a lower goal INR may be recommended

- Purple toe syndrome rarely happens likely to the patient being started on too high of an initial dose of warfarin
- Normal GI bacteria also produce vitamin K, changes in the gut bacteria due to antibiotics can also impact the INR

Xanthine Oxidase Inhibitors

Example: Allopurinol (Zyloprim), Febuxostat (Uloric)

Mechanism of Action: Inhibits xanthine oxidase and decreases uric acid production

NAPLEX Nuggets:

- Mechanism of Action: Common Uses: Decrease uric acid in gout
- Memorable Side Effects: GI issues, rash
- Used for prophylaxis of gout, NOT treatment of an acute flare; NSAIDs, prednisone, or colchicine are generally used for an acute flare
- Usually fairly well tolerated, but watch out for dose adjustments in CKD (allopurinol); cleared by the kidneys
- Keep an eye out for medications that can elevate uric acid; niacin, thiazide diuretics
- Febuxostat generally not first line as expensive $$ at this time

Did you find this review beneficial, if so please leave a kind review on Amazon! – Thanks in advance, Eric Christianson, PharmD

Made in the USA
Coppell, TX
06 June 2020

27149653R00098